A 3-DAY GUT CLEANSE

CANDI MCGRICA

CONTENTS

MEDICAL DISCLAIMER

The information in this book is intended for educational purpose only. It doesn't substitute any form of diagnosis, treatment, or medical advice. Always seek medical advisors regarding your health conditions. The author and the publisher are not held responsible for any consequences that result in applying information in this book.

INTRODUCTION

The stomach is the seat of all feeling. The heart is the seat of the conscience. The mind is the seat of the ego. Your body is the seat of the soul. When a man goes out in the night and looks up at the universe, he is observing a mirror of himself. The universe within us is a reflection of the universe we see out our eyes.

— SUZY KASSEM, *RISE UP AND SALUTE THE SUN: THE WRITINGS OF SUZY KASSEM*

Did you know that your gut is also your second mind (Pattemore, 2020)? It can be worried or relaxed and bears the effects of stress just like any other part of your body. Chronic stress is unbelievably the primary cause of digestive diseases in the United States (Bodybio, n.d.). And there is a reason for that: Stress disturbs the nervous system which negatively affects the gut system. And it works the other way: If your gut suffers, your whole well-being suffers as well. An unhealthy gut reflects on the outside. What's more, digestive problems are uncomfortable and tend to stay longer if you have no clue about the treatment. Besides, it's often difficult to determine at what moment you have to take them seriously. After all, constipation or an upset stomach can come and go with the help of some supplements. Sometimes, it feels like what you are eating doesn't really impact your digestion, right? After all, if your bowel movements are quite normal, it means that your gut is functional. Nevertheless, if you look closely, there might be many facts you ignore about your digestive health. One of them is your diet. Poor diet does have a direct correlation with your gut. Gas, diarrhea, constipation, and other inflammation result from eating a lot of processed food. Keep in mind that gut and fast food are enemies. Don't worry, I won't tell you to change your diet yet. If you love processed food, that's okay. The key is to balance your diet, your exercise, and your mental health.

But before that, there is a way to remedy your gut health, and it's a gut-cleanse process in which you have the chance to get rid of toxins and food intolerances. Through the R.E.S.T.O.R.E method, you will know more about your body's reactions to certain types of food to help you choose the best diet for yourself and improve your gut on the way. Most importantly, you will finally discover what's good and what's bad for your gut. Thanks to this 3-day investment, you can prevent many health problems for the years to come. Irritable Bowel Syndrome (IBS) and Inflammatory Bowel Disease (IBD) will finally disappear from your life as you will change your lifestyle.

Moreover, chronic gut problems go beyond your digestive health as they can lead to serious diseases such as diabetes, obesity, and heart diseases. Fortunately, it's not too late to aim for the flourishing gut and prevent these issues. For that reason, it's important to learn about the lively microbes living in your digestive system. It focuses on understanding the truth about how the environment and your lifestyle can enhance or endanger your gut microbiota. Therefore, change starts with awareness of these factors. The R.E.S.T.O.R.E method starts with eliminating food intolerances and toxins from your gut. You will then add new certain types of food to your diet to effectively remove those harmful elements from your body. Next, you will continue with the restoration phase, in which you implement gut-friendly food to diversify and promote your gut health. In the last step, you will be reintroduced to normal foods in small steps. At this stage, you will have to listen to your body and be aware of any changes that may occur, such as food intolerances, allergies, skin rashes, etc. To achieve the best outcomes from this process, you will have to transform your lifestyle. It consists of selecting the right food, optimizing your sleeping time, staying hydrated each day, and practicing physical exercises. Don't worry, in the last part of this book, you will learn how to adopt such a lifestyle to gain long-term benefits for your gut and your overall well-being.

The R.E.S.T.O.R.E method will set you on the right path to healing from gut diseases and preventing chronic diseases. To transform your well-being, you will discover the benefits of food supplements and the best way to include them in your diet. Probiotics and prebiotics are your best ally to support your gut system. You can start with natural food supplements to meet your recommended daily intake. If it seems difficult to you, at the end of each chapter, there will be a guide to plan your gut-friendly shopping list and meal plan. Nevertheless, what if you want to make a treat from time to time but still maintain your gut health? Then, you can rely on detoxifying foods as they are easy to prepare and can remove toxins and harmful elements from your body. Yet, they help to nurture your digestion and reduce inflammation. With the help of digestive enzymes, you can gain from natural foods and supplements, your body will be able to process food easily and break down nutrients so that you are strong, healthy, and still in good shape. Talking about your physical body, did you know that some exercises can trigger your gut and stimulate your gut system for better health? Through the brain-gut-muscle connection, there are a variety of exercises you can start in the comfort of your home, and you can get instant results and changes through regular practice. With a step-by-step guide, you will have the choice between different yoga poses. And if you've never practiced yoga before, these are completely beginner friendly. Some of these can be done in a few minutes, and before you eat your meal, so it's a win-win for your gut and your time.

In the last part of this book, we'll finally tackle stress to eradicate its effects on your physical health and optimize your mental state along the way. Stress does cause disturbance for your gut, but it is possible to stop it and change the way you manage it. You have the power to handle stress and overthinking in the simplest way possible by taking breathing exercises. Yes, you don't have to invest long hours a day to reduce stress in your life. A few minutes a day can help you to feel relaxed and peaceful each day. The good thing about these techniques is you can get instant benefits and practice them wherever you have the time. Breathing techniques do help to restore your peace of mind and reduce stress for a matter of a few minutes a day.

Regarding a gut-friendly lifestyle, balance and consistency are important. Whether it's about exercising, meditating, or breathing exercises, you reap the benefits of your efforts and investments through regular practice. If that seems daunting to you, the last chapter of this book is dedicated to helping you implement a gut-friendly lifestyle to achieve everlasting changes and gut health. In other words, you will enjoy all the benefits of being healthy and happier while taking good care of your gut. In fact, your well-being doesn't have to be a challenging day-to-day effort anymore. By choosing what works the best for you, whether it's your favorite detoxifying foods or your daily exercises, you can be free of any inflammation or digestive problems. And that's what this book gives to you: the choice. You have the choice of knowing what works and what doesn't. You have the choice to be aware of the power of better eating for your life. You don't have to wait for tomorrow to change your life. All you must do is learn what you need to know about your gut and enjoy the adventure of a gut-friendly lifestyle. So, what you'll read next will give you all the information you need to know to understand how your gut works and why a better understanding of your gut system will give you clarity and mastery about your physical well-being. So, keep reading because everything about your gut will be revealed to start your gut-friendly journey.

STEP 1: PREPARATION

1

GUT INSTINCTS

Understanding your gut is the door to making the huge leap toward your goals. Whether you are looking to lose weight or seeking to improve your well-being and feel good in your skin, taking the time to learn about your gut will make a difference. In fact, by having in mind the system behind your gut, you will come to assimilate new information faster and make your journey more fascinating and life-changing. So, what does a 3-day gut cleanse do to your body exactly? Well, not only does it aim to better your gut health, but it also helps to switch to a more healthful diet. Therefore, if you want to change your well-being, you should start by enhancing the number of good bacteria in your gut. A gut cleanse is then the path to effectively improve your gut health through a meticulous process.

It encompasses being familiar with how the gut functions so that you can easily implement new habits in your diet. A 3-day gut cleanse consists of removing harmful bacteria from your gut and making a place for beneficial bacteria. Most importantly, it comes with a new healthy lifestyle to achieve long-term benefits. But, before starting the R.E.S.T.O.R.E method, understanding how your gut functions is the key to successfully adopting new changes in your life.

WHAT DOES THE GUT DO?

It may seem surprising, but the digestive system is not just about the stomach. The mouth, the esophagus, the stomach, the small and large intestines, the rectum, and the anus are all part of the digestive system. It means that all these parts of the body participate in digestion. That's why, from the moment you eat, your gut is exposed to the good as well as the bad bacteria from your food. You have more control over your gut than you've ever imagined. How it works might be invisible to your eyes, but you can influence the way it functions to enhance your well-being. And as you will soon discover in this chapter, your gut is considered as a brain as well. Most of the body's immune cells are also produced in the gut. It also yields healthy metabolites and shelters 95% of serotonin (Danone Research, n.d.).

WHAT IS GUT HEALTH?

The gut microbiome, composed of trillions of microbes stored in the gut, ensures the digestive system, and metabolizes nutrients the body needs to stay alive. Probiotics are healthy bacteria. With enough probiotics, you can fight unhealthy bacteria in the gut. Probiotics come from natural foods and supplements. Prebiotics maintain the vitality of good bacteria and can be found in fermented foods such as kombucha, pickles, and in yogurt.

Not only does the gut ensure the digestive system, but it also supports overall health. For example, the gut is important for immune function, preventing viruses and fungi from entering the bloodstream (Mudge, 2022). *A leaky gut* happens when the gut is vulnerable due to different factors such as diet and antibiotic intake. Common signs of digestive problems are bloating, constipation, and nausea. Fatigue, poor sleep, and bad breath are also signals of gut problems. Did you know that your gut health condition starts at birth? The moment you were born, you were exposed to bacteria through birth delivery and maternal conditions (Mudge, 2022). Apart from genetics, the environment and lifestyle also affect the gut.

WHY IS GUT HEALTH IMPORTANT?

A healthy gut equals a balance between good bacteria and bad bacteria (Everlywell, 2022). If your digestive system isn't working properly, this will result in a weak immune system and bad digestion. The gut helps to remove toxins from your body. Stress, poor nutrition, and overuse of antibiotics are harmful to gut health (Everlywell, 2022). If you want to know if you have a healthy gut, first, notice your bowel movements. If they are regular and don't take effort and pain, it is a good sign. Also, notice how often you experience bloating. There are also other factors such as your reactions to stress, how you feel energized during the day—which means you have taken the right nutrition to help digestion—and your ability to concentrate. Make sure you have fiber-rich food in your diet to revitalize your gut. Try to minimize processed food and overconsumption as well.

THE GUT-BRAIN CONNECTION

The gut and brain are strongly related. The gut is called the *second brain* or Enteric Nervous System (ENS) (Harvard Health Publishing, 2019). The ENS can cause emotional problems for people experiencing functional bowel problems such as diarrhea, constipation, bloating, stomach upset, pain, and stomach upset. Antidepressants and mind-body therapies such as Cognitive behavioral therapy (CBT) are proven to be effective as they act on nerve cells in the gut (Johns Hopkins Medicine, 2019). CBT plays a role in improving communication between the two brains.

In daily life, the brain and gut interfere with each other. For example, the sight of a juice provokes a reaction in your gut, while a clenching gut occurs at the fear of being late for a job interview. What's more, stomach pain can be the cause or the result of stress as well. Anxiety is proven to worsen the symptoms of Irritable Bowel Syndrome (IBS) or Inflammatory Bowel Disease (IBD) (Harvard Health Publishing, 2019). According to a study, the majority of patients with Crohn's disease assert that stressful circumstances affect their disease (Kinsinger, 2017). Besides, stress can induce gastrointestinal disease as gut nerves are sensitive to respond to stress symptoms.

MAINTAINING A HEALTHY GUT MICROBIOME

What is the Gut Microbiome?

Also called microbiota, the gut microbiome encompasses trillions of healthy and unhealthy microbes inside the body (Harvard Health Publishing, 2019). It includes bacteria, viruses, and fungi that are coexisting together. To understand it clearly, picture the gut microbiome as an entire entity ensuring the good function of the digestive system. But as you will see later, the gut microbiome can impact your overall health and not just your digestive health.

Why is It Crucial for Your Health?

The gut microbiome can affect your health positively or negatively. Good bacteria protect you from any harm, whereas bad bacteria are dangerous for your gut health. For example, studies have found that the gut microbiome—the friendly bacteria—supports good cholesterol and decreases the risk of heart disease. Besides, it helps to manage blood sugar and prevent the risks of diabetes.

An imbalance of gut microbiome—bad bacteria dominate over good bacteria— is the root of many diseases. It weakens the immune system and spreads toxins all over your body. And that's how the body becomes vulnerable to diseases.

How Does Microbiota Benefit the Body?

Microbiota is beneficial for the body thanks to its different roles in the digestive system. By helping to digest certain types of fiber, it contributes to the creation of short-chain fatty acids, which helps to prevent many diseases such as cancer and cardiovascular diseases. It also interferes with different parts of your health, such as your weight, your brain health, and chronic diseases. Microbiota is a whole population of microbes living in your gut system, mainly in the small and large intestines and throughout the body. It's important to note that the gut microbiome is vulnerable. Different factors can damage good bacteria. For example, poor diet, chronic stress, and antibiotics overuse can all disturb the composition of your gut microbiome.

Thanks to the help of microbiota, the body can break down vitamins for its vitality. What's more, sugars are absorbed in the small intestine, but only the microbiota can help to break them down with digestive enzymes (Harvard Health Publishing, 2019). Thanks to its influence on the immune system, the microbiota helps to prevent infection. Besides, it helps to control weight as the more balanced your gut microbiome is, the more it contributes to minimizing the risk of obesity and keeping a balanced weight. Apart from that, the gut microbiome can positively reduce the risk of heart disease by increasing good cholesterol (Harvard Health Publishing, 2019). And thanks to the existence of a healthy bacteria called *Lactobacilli*, the gut microbiome can effectively help to lower bad cholesterol. Finally, the microbiota can enhance your brain health by promoting serotonin, an antidepressant neurotransmitter that is produced in the gut (Harvard Health Publishing, 2019).

Can Diet Affect One's Microbiota?

The food you eat contains elements that influence the composition and diversity of your gut microbiota. Particularly, specific foods such as probiotics contain lively bacteria, which is helpful for your gut. Probiotics include fermented foods such as kefir, kombucha, and sauerkraut. Natural foods such as legumes, fruits, and vegetables can promote the microbiota as they serve as food for the good bacteria, helping in their growth and diversity. Most importantly, the more variety of food you have in your diet, the healthier your microbiota will become. High-fiber foods such as whole grains also contain prebiotics which are excellent gut-friendly food. Certain types of food rich in polyphenols also support the growth of good bacteria in the gut. These can be found in red wine, green tea, and dark chocolate. Lastly, food supplements such as probiotics and prebiotics can be helpful in balancing your gut microbiota.

THE IMPORTANCE OF HYDRATION FOR YOUR GUT

Water keeps the body hydrated, but is it beneficial for the gut in some ways? Hydration aids the body in removing waste through perspiration, urination, and defecation. Enough hydration means that the body can regulate fluids. Moreover, water supports the gut system by preventing constipation, according to researchers at the University of Rochester Medical Center (University of Rochester, 2019). Most importantly, hydration is crucial for digestion in different ways. For example, it contributes to the digestion of some types of fiber and helps the body to break down nutrients. What's more, more water can impact the function of the large intestine by transforming stools from liquid to solid. Some research also suggests that hydration can play an important role in the vitality of the gut microbiome by promoting the right condition for the gut flora (Migala, 2015). Eating fruits can help you stay hydrated as well so that you don't have to drink water all day long.

INSIGHT INTO YOUR GUT HEALTH

The following guide will help you understand your gut in a better way and serves as a premise to implement your gut-friendly lifestyle.

- What types of food make me feel good after eating them?

- What are the foods that seem to hurt my gut?

- How would I rate my gut health and why?

- Do I have some signs of an unhealthy gut? What are they?

- Am I ready to follow an elimination diet to better my gut health?

- What foods do I usually eat that are good for my gut health?

- What types of food can I try to include in my meal plan to diversify my diet and improve my gut health?

- What foods have impacted my mood and my mind lately?

- How can better gut health change my well-being and my life?

- What could be the factors that prevent me from having a healthier gut?

Your gut health matters. Not only does it ensure the function of your digestive system, but it also supports your overall well-being. In fact, it is interdependent on your mental health, thanks to the gut-brain connection. To foster your gut health, managing stress is important to limit inflammation and other digestive diseases. Moreover, aiming to obtain a healthy gut is feasible thanks to your diet, which plays an important role in the growth of your gut microbiome. However, an imbalanced diet based on processed food is harmful to the lively bacteria in the gut as it provokes an imbalance between the good and the bad microbes. In addition to that, it can cause several digestive problems, such as: gas, bloating, diarrhea, constipation, and chronic diseases, such as diabetes. Therefore, it's important to be aware of the different factors that could harm your gut. In the next chapter, you will achieve a deep understanding of the different factors that are disastrous for your gut. Such knowledge will contribute to a better gut-friendly lifestyle and aids in preventing chronic diseases. Furthermore, understanding the reality behind processed food and how it affects your gut will give an insight into the importance of the 3-day gut-cleanse method to improve your gut health and help you reach your health goals.

2

GOODBYE, INFLAMMATION

Are you tired of experiencing ingrained pain that seems unimportant, yet it makes you feel uncomfortable? Some of these painful states are fatigue, skin problems, and abdominal pain. More often, you look for a remedy that soothes the pain, but it doesn't take it away. Let me tell you something: Your gut has more effects on your overall health than you've ever imagined. When your gut is unhealthy, your health suffers as well.

Let's find out the different signals of an unhealthy gut you should pay attention to. Above all, there are common symptoms related to your digestive system. They are easier to recognize, such as constipation, bloating, abdominal pain, and diarrhea. When you experience any of these, know that there is an imbalance of gut bacteria in your gastrointestinal system, which results in IBS. It means your gut doesn't function in a normal way because there are not enough good bacteria. It could be explained by your diet or the medicine you take, such as antibiotics. But as you will see later, there are tremendous and somehow unbelievable factors of an imbalanced gut.

What about fatigue? Have you ever felt exhausted despite taking a rest? From now on, be aware of your gut when you feel tired, especially if it's frequent, because the presence of bad bacteria in your gut can induce a feeling of exhaustion (Nagy-Szakal et al., 2017). I know, your gut may not be the first thing that comes to your mind when you feel tired. And you can't reject other factors according to your circumstances, but it's helpful to know that unexplained fatigue is one of the symptoms of an unhealthy gut. Such a piece of knowledge can avoid waste of time and money and helps to prevent and remedy the symptom effectively.

Skin problems and food intolerances are related to gut problems as well. Researchers have found that unfriendly gut microbiome can accumulate in the skin through your bloodstream, which results in destroying the skin homeostasis (Nagy-Szakal et al., 2017). What's more, the gut can also "influence the cutaneous defense mechanisms" (Nagy-Szakal et al., 2017). Regarding food intolerances, gut imbalance can potentially bring about respiratory, cutaneous, and food allergies. Unfavorable nutrition and environment can harm the gut, which then causes disorders in the immune response, but also the skin and lung microbiome.

Finally, chronic depression and anxiety can be the cause of the result of gut disturbance. In distressing situations, both your brain and your gut can *undergo* stress in some psychological and physical ways. For example, you can feel nauseated because of fear.

GUT BACTERIA AND DISEASES

Gut bacteria play different roles in the organism, particularly the gut system. Before expounding on the disastrous effects of bad bacteria and how it causes diseases, let's discover the different benefits of gut microbiota for gut function. The gut bacteria have multiple roles in the gut system. For example, gut bacteria are responsible for refueling essential nutrients for the body. It also helps to absorb minerals. Besides, gut bacteria shelter the gut defense system as a protection against the invasion of pathogenic bacteria and supports the host immune system (Zhang et al., 2015). Moreover, gut bacteria help to eliminate toxins and contribute to the metabolism of isoflavones, an important element in reducing the risk of breast cancer, prostate cancer, cardiovascular disease, osteoporosis, and menopausal symptoms (Zhang et al., 2015).

Abnormal changes are fatal for the gut system as they lead to dysfunction and imbalance in the gut bacteria. When the gut is oversaturated by harmful bacteria, the gut flora becomes vulnerable to diseases (Zhang et al., 2015). For instance, the excessive intake of antibiotics destroys good bacteria. Consequently, when there aren't enough healthy bacteria, the body struggles to fight against the effects of bad bacteria. It means that an imbalance in the gut composition is the main cause of Inflammatory Bowel Diseases. What's more, research has proven that gut imbalance has a correlation with diseases such as obesity, diabetes, liver diseases, chronic heart diseases, and cancer (Zhang et al., 2015). A dietary fat diet affects the bacteria composition as it increases the ratio of bacteria responsible for body weight. It influences obesity by "promoting chronic inflammatory status" (Zhang et al., 2015). Moreover, gut imbalance contributes to diabetes as it promotes the increase of insulin resistance, the cause of type-2 diabetes. Lastly, the presence of harmful bacteria contributes to the development of gastrointestinal cancer and prostate cancer.

WHAT HARMS YOUR GUT

Physical Things That Harm Your Gut Bacteria

Nutrition can maintain and harm gut bacteria. A balanced gut flora means a healthier gut microbiome and less unhealthy bacteria. It means that your gut microbiome is lively and functional in supporting your gut system. To nurture those friendly bacteria, it's important to know the reasons behind gut imbalance. First, an unvaried diet and a lack of prebiotics from fiber don't contribute to the growth of good bacteria. In fact, fiber is an important ingredient that supports gut health as it contains prebiotics, the elements which propel the growth and maintenance of healthy bacteria. Fiber is mainly found in fruits and vegetables. Eating too much protein intake, particularly factory-farmed meat, is unhealthy because it can increase the harmful bacteria in the gut system. Furthermore, refined sugar and processed food can result in constipation and metabolic diseases as they bring about negative effects on the gut microbiome. Dairies are also known as the cause of inflammation and intestinal diseases.

Second, antibiotics are dangerous for the gut micro-biota for several reasons. One of them is the decrease in the diversity of microbes living in the gut because of these antibiotics. They prevent good bacteria from growing. They also increase antibiotic resistance, responsible for nearly 35,000 deaths in the United States and 25,000 deaths in Europe each year (*The Bacterial Challenge: Time to React a Call to Narrow the Gap between Multidrug-Resistant Bacteria in the EU and the Development of New Antibacterial Agents*, n.d.). Antibiotic resistance causes serious infections whose treatment is costly and challenging. Most importantly, the presence of antibiotics in the diet and antibiotic overuse simply kills the good bacteria in the gut system.

Apart from the imbalanced microbiome, excessive alcohol leads to a leaky gut, a state in which the gut becomes less resistant to toxins and bad bacteria. Alcohol also damages the liver by gathering fats which potentially leads to fatty liver diseases such as cancer or cirrhosis. What's more, it affects other parts of the digestive system causing serious inflammation in the pancreas. Cigarette smoking can negatively impact the gut microbiome as well, causing intestinal disorders associated with celiac disease and colorectal cancer.

Psychological Factors

Stress creates physical reactions in your body, particularly in your gut. Common results of stress include nausea and loss of appetite. Depending on one person to another, stress does disturb your digestive health in different ways. For instance, when you feel in danger or if a situation seems scary to you, it may result in losing your appetite. Because of the fight-or-flight response, the body releases the stress hormone cortisol (Iliades, 2018). The latter set off different reactions to the gut system by increasing the acid in the stomach, which causes indigestion. But when stress becomes frequent, it can aggravate IBS such as diarrhea and constipation. Hence, stress—whether you feel angry, sad, or depressed—is more closely related to your digestive health than you can ever imagine. And one way to enhance your gut health is by reducing stress as much as you can. Fortunately, different exercises can help in minimizing the effects of stress, which we'll develop later in this book.

Sleep deprivation is a mental condition that negatively impacts the gut flora as well. A lack of sleep could worsen overthinking and negativity in a stressful situation. Yet, when the body experiences tension and mental strains, the gut system becomes vulnerable to inflammation, stomach pain, and food sensitivities. Moreover, a lack of sleep can affect your diet and eating habits, as emotions can increase your appetite and influence your food choices accordingly. Most importantly, sleep deprivation can increase the bacteria responsible for weight gain, obesity, type 2 diabetes, and fat metabolism. Hence, make sure you have enough sleep to lower the risk of digestive issues and ease your digestion daily.

FOODS TO AVOID

Processed Food

Processed food includes fast food, manufactured snacks and biscuits, and pastries. These are tasty and quite affordable, made from excessive salt, sugar, vegetable oils, animal fat, and flour. They are also available everywhere and addictive. The more people are used to eating processed food, the less they are inclined to opt for a healthier and fiber-rich diet. Yet, processed food does harm the gut and overall health. According to researchers, the presence of food additives in highly processed food can alter the gut microbiota, causing bowel issues, inflammatory diseases, food intolerances, and even autoimmune conditions (Zinöcker & Lindseth, 2018). For example, having less fiber in the diet, even for a matter of a few days, increases the risk of constipation.

Besides, an unvaried diet can develop the risk of getting food intolerance. Eating the same types of food leads to indigestion and makes it difficult for your digestive system to absorb nutrients properly. Common food intolerances are lactose, which is related to dairy products such as milk, histamine contained in pineapple, chocolate, bananas, and gluten, found in wheat, rye, and barley.

What's more, processed foods are devoid of the essential nutrients the body needs to fight diseases. More often, they contain excessive salt, sugar, and food additives. They also lack probiotics and prebiotics, which are mainly essential for gut health.

Artificial Sweeteners and the Gut Microbiota

The variants of artificial sweeteners are *sucralose, sorbitol, mannitol, erythritol,* and *aspartame* (Aliouche, 2022). Used as a replacement for real sugar, they lack energy intake and are simply used to sweeten and flavor food. More often, they are present in processed food. There are two types of sweeteners. The first one is non-nutritive, which has lower calories and is used for its taste. The second one is low-calorie sweeteners. Examples include polyols or sugar alcohols. They are low-digestible carbohydrates produced from hydrogenating sugar or syrup.

When it comes to the gut system, sugar and artificial sweeteners do more harm than good to the gut microbiota. In fact, they have direct effects on the gut microbiota as they cause disturbance to the composition of gut microbes. Besides, they mainly cause glucose intolerance. It's important to note that the gut microbiota is responsible for metabolism, immunity, anabolism, and cognitive function and enhances the development of immune cells (Aliouche, 2022). By directly attacking the gut microbiota, artificial sweeteners can bring serious health issues. A change in metabolism, weight gain, and metabolic disturbance are some of the consequences of gut microbiota disturbance.

Gluten and Leaky Gut

Gluten is a protein that can be found in grains like wheat, barley, and rye. It's interesting to know that gluten can particularly enhance intestinal permeability, also called leaky gut syndrome. In fact, gluten can enlarge the gaps between the cells in the small intestine because it influences *zonulin*, an element responsible for intestinal permeability (Bell, 2016). In the case of leaky gut syndrome, the gut microbiota becomes vulnerable to toxins and other harmful bacteria. Imagine those cells serve as a barrier to toxins. When they become permeable, toxins have access to the overall organism, which leads to inflammation (Bell, 2016). When inflammation becomes persistent, there are risks for chronic diseases such as diabetes and obesity. Furthermore, gluten intolerance can induce celiac disease and hereditary autoimmune disease.

NEW HABITS FOR SAYING GOODBYE TO INFLAMMATION FOR GOOD

- Add more colors to your meals. Do you struggle to find ideas for your meals and end up grabbing fast food instead? The secret to making healthy meal choices is to add more colors to your diet. Natural foods such as green leafy vegetables, berries, grapes, bananas, carrots, etc., can make your diet more appealing and enhance your gut health. Besides, the more varied your food choices are, the lesser the risk of inflammation. To optimize your gut health, start with varying your main course and dessert each day. Planning your meal plan every week can be helpful to get more ideas on what to eat next. Whenever you have new ideas for your meal, take notes and add them to your plan.
- Make a treat for yourself once a week. You don't have to deprive yourself of processed food. The key is to eat them as rarely as possible in a week or a month. And if you ever feel like a juicy burger is the only thing your palate craves, don't be guilty. Remedy the situation by increasing your fiber intake the next day.
- Sleep, sleep, sleep. You don't have to increase your sleeping time. All you have to do is to go

to bed at the same hour and keep the same duration of sleep each night. Avoiding caffeine intake in the afternoon and trying to eat at least two hours before bed can help you to find sleep easily. What's more, you can try to reduce your screen time before bed to help you sleep well at night.

- Replace your snacks with fruits. If eating healthy food might be challenging at the beginning, you can replace your snacks with fruits instead. There's no better rule than prioritizing what you love to eat first. You can be creative by making a smoothie, eating dried fruits from time to time, or trying other fruits you are not used to eating as a dessert, for example.

- Dedicate time for self-care each day. Having a few minutes a day for yourself is important to better manage your mood and emotions. Try to have time for yourself where you get your mind off your occupation. You can spend time doing nothing, taking a walk, getting a massage, listening to music, reading, or just breathing. Those simple habits can then be transformed into stress-relief moments once you replace them with meditation and other mindfulness

exercises, which you will learn later in this
book.

Your gut system supports your well-being. When it's
clear that factors such as stress and processed food are
harmful to your gut microbiome, it's much easier to
make changes. More often, an unvaried diet leads to a
lack of fiber intake and overconsumption of processed
food. Fortunately, it's possible to improve your gut and
reduce inflammation for good. Thanks to simple habits,
you can start to make small changes. In the next chapters, you will gain more practical tips on how to
enhance your gut health. You'll be introduced to the
R.E.S.T.O.R.E method to finally start your gut-cleanse
journey. You will learn the best foods to optimize your
gut from toxins. This step is helpful if you have some
weight-loss goals as well.

3

FEEDING THE GARDEN WITHIN

The R.E.S.T.O.R.E method is a gut-cleanse process that aims to revitalize gut health. Similar to the detox method, it mainly focuses on creating a flourishing digestive health regardless of your age and your background relationship with diet. This method works best, especially if you want to shift to a lifestyle change. It is extremely beneficial if you have used different ways to lose weight but didn't achieve satisfying results in the long-term. In fact, it helps you to consider your diet in a positive way and revamp the way you think about food and diet in general. So, it starts with the elimination phase. This stage is very important because it will set you on the right path to cleaning your gut. It is mainly based on the best foods that help to detoxify and purge your body from toxins you've accumulated over the years. It is essentially a huge step to renew your digestive system and to gain a new perspective on your gut. It is a positive way to heal your gut and an introduction to a gut-friendly lifestyle. The second step, which is the restoration phase, consists of nourishing your gut with the right food. Again, not all foods are beneficial for your digestive health. Therefore, it's always important to remember the goal, which is to restore your gut in order to be healthier and have a balanced weight. The foods that are suggested in this method are essential for your health goals as well. For example, fiber is an excellent food for the gut, and if you want to lose weight, eating a high-fiber diet will help you to manage your appetite. So, keep in mind that a gut-cleanse method is a powerful way to foster your overall well-being. What's more, the R.E.S.T.O.R.E doesn't stop there. It also assists you in reintroducing other types of food step-by-step so that the change doesn't come so abrupt for your gut. Yet, you can still benefit from this gut-cleanse journey while fueling your body with nutrients. Remember, when it comes to food, balance is the key. Choosing the right foods for your gut will give you more freedom to balance your diet in a way that suits you the most. As you will see in the next chapters of this book, there are different ways to make this journey perfect and beneficial for yourself in the long term.

UNDERSTANDING THE PHASE OF THE GUT CLEANSE

Day 1: Elimination Phase

Understanding the Elimination Phase

This first day consists of inserting gut-friendly food that contributes to eliminating toxins from your organism. The goal is to restore your gut health from scratch by using specific detox foods. It will help to determine food sensitivities, intolerances, and allergies as well. The elimination phase yields tremendous benefits for the gut and well-being. A key meal plan helps to understand gut health and how the body reacts to certain types of food. Food sensitivities occur when there is an imbalance of gut microbiomes in the gastrointestinal system. As gut health is dependent on your diet, this step aids in finding the best meal plan that is favorable to your gut microbiota. It's important to take notes of the different changes that occur during the phase. For instance, keep track of the reactions to certain types of food that you might be unfamiliar with.

What's more, it serves as an assessment to choose the best diet regardless of your health goals. Based on gut-friendly food, the elimination phase considers the process of healing and repairing your gut from gastrointestinal issues such as bloating, diarrhea, and so forth. Besides, this is a key step to find out if the body has enough digestive enzymes, which are important to dispose of certain sugars.

Three Rules for a Successful Elimination Phase

- Keep your diet simple. Simplicity is the secret to unlocking your journey to a successful and healthy gut cleanse. As a matter of fact, keep track of the types of foods that you need to prioritize and aim to have them in each of your meal plans. Most importantly, focus on choosing fresh foods that are healthier for your gut. As you will see later on, you have lots of choices when it comes to eating healthy. Always try to prioritize fiber-rich food and gut-soothing food such as bananas, spinach, and fruit juice. These are your best ally to transform your health and achieve any health goals you've always aimed for. Whether you're trying to lose weight or improve your digestive health, these types of food won't disappoint you.
- Remove inflammatory food from your diet. You know what? The simplest way to nurture your gut is to get rid of all the physical factors that cause inflammation. Some of them are processed food, refined sugar, and hydrogenated oils. In this journey, you will

learn to adopt a new diet for yourself to gain all the benefits of eating healthy while solving all your digestive problems. Hence, learn to replace inflammatory foods with the ones that are best for your gut. Key foods are your best ally to regenerate your digestive health and eliminate inflammation for good.

- Reduce stress to favor the gut-brain connection. It's important to handle stress to avoid digestive problems. As this journey aims to restore your gut health, learn to avoid stress by getting enough sleep, for example. Focus on having quality sleep and try to manage your mood. Don't hesitate to take a break to breathe and get relaxed to minimize the effects of stressful situations on your mind. What's more, learn to prioritize your emotional well-being. You can manage negative emotions such as anger, resentment, revenge, and anxiety by shifting your mood to a positive one. In this journey, cherish all the benefits you'll get from adopting a new diet and eating new and healthier types of food. The R.E.S.T.O.R.E method is, above all, a positive perspective to restore your well-being from the effects of toxins and stress. Therefore, be optimistic and boost your mood with positive emotions such as gratitude, well-being, and peace of mind.

Key Foods and Supplements for Day 1

Firstly, let's start with the types of food that you should ban from your diet on this first day: wheat-based products. Examples include bread, pasta, cereals, and wheat flour. Baked goods and snacks should be excluded as well. These are cakes, muffins, pizza, crackers, pretzels, potato chips, and candy bars. Gluten-based food such as barley, rye, bulgur, and seitan shouldn't be included. Most importantly, don't use artificial sweeteners and refined oils such as sunflower and soybean. For beverages, alcohol, and sugary drinks such as soda should be avoided as well.

Secondly, let's focus on the best gut-friendly food you need to include in your diet. Start with prioritizing vegetables that contribute to improving gut health. You have the choices between broccoli, cauliflower, Brussels sprouts, cabbage, arugula, carrots, kale, beetroot, all leafy greens, celery, cucumber, peas, radishes, Swiss chard, spinach, ginger, mushrooms, and zucchini. Next, include healthy sources of fat such as coconut oil, olive oil, nuts, seed, avocado oil, and avocados. Gluten-free grains are also beneficial for you. These are buckwheat, amaranth, rice (brown and white), sorghum, teff, and gluten-free oats. To add a taste to your meal, you can include all herbs and spices. If you want to opt for fish on some days, try to prioritize salmon, tuna, herring, and other omega-3-rich fish. Some food is extremely beneficial for gut health. There are fermented vegetables like kimchi, sauerkraut, tempeh, and miso, along with cultured dairy products such as kefir, yogurt, Greek yogurt, and traditional buttermilk.

Lastly, regarding fruits, you have the choice between coconut, grapes, bananas, blueberries, raspberries, strawberries, kiwi, pineapple, oranges, mandarin, lemon, limes, passionfruit, and papaya. These are all good for digestion. As for beverages, you can opt for bone broth, teas, coconut milk, nut milk, water, and kombucha. Nuts, including peanuts, almonds, and nut milks, are in your favor as well.

A Sample Meal Plan for Day 1

For breakfast, there are different meal plans you can alternate. Keep in mind that these are simple suggestions, but you can opt for different types of food from the recommended key foods above.

- Option 1: Banana and blueberries accompanied with Greek yogurt and unsweetened almond milk. Bananas are perfect for breakfast. It is excellent for digestive health and is a 100% gut-friendly food. Combined with bananas, eating blueberries and Greek yogurt is the best way to start your day and optimize your gut.

- Option 2: Omelet with vegetables of your choice and avocado. This is a simple meal to have vegetables in your breakfast. Yet, you have the choice of ingredients to prepare a tasty and gut-friendly meal. Don't forget to add avocado to fuel your body with healthy nutrients. In fact, avocado oil is one of the best ingredients for health as well.

- Option 3: Mushroom, spinach, and zucchini frittata. Are you keen on energizing your gut with a high-fiber diet? If the answer is yes, then option 3 is the best choice for you. Inspired by the recipe published by the food blog *Eating Well*, you can prepare your frittata by preheating your broiler and beating your eggs before cooking to get a consistent and non-watery egg (Eating Well, 2020). Don't hesitate to use extra-virgin olive oil and add fresh mint and fresh basil for flavors.

For lunch, you can choose from the following meal plan.

- Option 1: Mixed green salad with sliced hard-boiled eggs. For a tasty green salad, the food blog Le Creme de la Crumb suggests a moderate variety of vegetables, such as green leaf lettuce, spinach, broccoli, cauliflower, kale, and avocado oil (Tiffany, 2019).
- Option 2: Chicken salad with olive oil. Chicken salad is easy to prepare. To have a lighter taste, try adding lemon juice, and don't forget to add pepper for seasoning. You can add some veggies, such as celery and parsley, to have some greens in your salad.
- Option 3: Sweet potato halves stuffed with spinach, turkey, and fresh cranberries. A tasty and low-calorie dinner, this is the best option if you want something other than salad for lunch.

For dinner, get inspired by the following options.

- Option 1: Beef and broccoli stir-fry with zucchini noodles and sauerkraut. This is a super easy meal for dinner and will give a feeling of fullness.

- Option 2: Seared salmon served with a fresh garden salad. Salmon is another light option for dinner. If you aren't keen on eating meat, this one is the perfect dinner for you.
- Option 3: Baked chicken served with roasted carrots, beans, and broccoli. Chicken combined with veggies is a perfect way to have a delicious dinner while getting enough fiber intake.

Keep in mind to vary your diet by using gut-friendly ingredients. The key is to add veggies, whole-grain foods, and vegetables, which are great sources of prebiotics in each of your meal plans. To flavor your meal, you can opt for gut-friendly herbs and spices such as ginger, basil, mint, cinnamon, and curry.

Day 2: Restoration Phase

Understanding the Restoration Phase

Once you've removed all toxins and other elements that cause disturbance to your gut flora, it's time to enhance and promote your gut microbiome with the right food (Lawrence & Hyde, 2017). This step is based on diversifying the good bacteria to establish a balanced and healthier gut. It mainly consists of taking probiotics and prebiotics. The former are sources of good bacteria, and the latter supports gut health by helping the growth of the gut microbiome. In addition to that, it's still important to influence your gut health in every manner by reducing stress, getting enough sleep, and doing exercises.

Nourishing the Gut

The essential thing is to minimize sugar and sweetener. As the goal is to diversify the good bacteria, try to reduce antibiotic intake. Finally, make sure to get enough sleep, make time for exercise, and limit stress by controlling your mood and your thoughts. As for diet, choosing a vegetarian diet can be a good idea during this phase.

Key Foods

Probiotics include yogurt, kefir, sauerkraut, kimchi, sourdough, almonds, and kombucha. Considered as *restoration* food, they help to revitalize and strengthen your gut health effectively. In this process, we prioritize natural sources of probiotics, but there will be more guidance about taking probiotics supplements later on in this book. Another key component of this step is feeding the gut with prebiotics. Prebiotics are undigested food that helps the gut microbiota to grow and function in the intestines. In other words, they are food for the good bacteria. Important sources of prebiotics are peas, Brussels sprouts, bananas, garlic, and ginger.

A Sample Meal Plan for Day 2

For breakfast, you can choose from the three alternatives below.

- Option 1: Kefir, banana, almond, and berry smoothie. This breakfast is easy to do and contains enough gut-friendly food to start the day.
- Option 2: Banana pancake and Greek Yogurt. This option is the best choice if you would love to feel full while having enough probiotics intake, as Greek yogurt is a great source of probiotics.
- Option 3: Blueberry smoothie. This smoothie is rich in antioxidants and supports the gut system. You can add crunchy granola and shaved coconut for a maximum of nutrients.

For lunch, feel free to get inspired by the following options.

- Option 1: Smoked salmon with avocado. This delicious lunch is rich in healthy fats and omega-3.
- Option 2: Miso soup with veggies. Rich in probiotics and prebiotics, this option will feed

your gut microbiome while supporting your digestive health.

- Option 3: Grain and veggie salad with tempeh. This is another 100% gut-friendly lunch. Try to prioritize whole grains for this lunch. As for veggies, choose what's tastier and more appealing to you. Tempeh is another source of probiotics for your gut.

For dinner, you can choose between these options.

- Option 1: Grilled chicken wings with raw carrots, celery, and sauerkraut. Chicken tastes well with carrots and celery. For a low-calorie dinner, pre-boil the chicken before grilling it.
- Option 2: Broiled steak with Brussels sprouts and sweet potatoes. Add salt, pepper, and steak seasoning to make this dinner tastier. 10 to 12 minutes is the best time to cook the steak with a high-heat broiler.
- Option 3: Green salad with chickpeas. With a combination of cucumber, Swiss cheese, and chickpeas, this is a light dinner without meat and could be served with some grilled vegetables.

Day 3: Reintroduction Phase

Understanding the Reintroduction Phase

This last step consists of making the transition from a gut-friendly diet to a normal diet in a step-by-step manner. It helps to reintroduce new food while taking care of your gut health. It starts with reintroducing the least inflammatory food. The key is to keep supporting your gut microbiome while making sure the reintroduction phase runs smoothly. Then, make sure to vary your introductory food while keeping your gut-friendly ingredients. Lastly, you can take processed food, but only in a small portion. Keep your main diet as gut-friendly as possible by having vegetables or fermented food, and don't forget to eat fruits even between your meal for snacks.

Reintroducing Foods

The reintroduction phase is a key step to switching to a healthier and gut-friendly diet for the long term. Your efforts during these two last days will eventually pay off by having a balanced diet. It means that you can start eating processed food and add refined sugar to your meal. However, you need to have your priority in mind —which is to support your gut microbiome through your new lifestyle. The reintroduction phase encompasses a few rules to follow. By taking these into account every day, you can successfully improve your gut health and your well-being and achieve your health goals.

- Choose the right time to practice the 3-day gut cleanse. It's important to get prepared ahead of time before embarking on this journey. If the reintroduction phase gets neglected, it would be a challenge to get started again. Yet, choosing the right type of food is essential for this last step. Therefore, ensure that you have everything you need and get prepared mentally to get the best outcomes. Besides, take the time to understand the process thoroughly. Also, make sure you are available to prepare your food at home and dedicate time to get away from stress.
- Pay attention to food reactions. Watch out for any changes or reactions that you may encounter. For example, take into consideration allergies and food intolerances once you start reintroducing processed food into your diet. Symptoms include diarrhea, skin rashes, itching or tingling lips, abdominal pain, gas, cramp, nausea, and vomiting (Mayo Clinic, 2017). When you experience reactions to a certain type of food, take notes of it. Keep in

mind that it's okay to have such a reaction after the elimination and restoration phases. That's why it's beneficial to start with the least inflammatory food first to reduce the risk of having serious food reactions, as a sudden change is likely to have impacts on your gut.

- Take small steps at a time. Don't rush to take fast food or processed food in this last step. Instead, you can either add refined sugar to your beverages or take a small portion of your favorite meal, for example. Choose wisely what you want to eat. Remember, heavily processed food doesn't go hand in hand with a probiotics-based diet. For example, you can opt for a small portion of a low-fiber or easy-to-digest food.

- Be mindful when you eat. This 3-day gut cleanse is a way to connect with yourself through the food you eat. It's a path to better understand your relationship with your food and the best time to listen to your body's reactions to the different types of food. Hence, take your time whenever you prepare your meal, take your meal, or when you choose to be attentive to your body's reactions to food. When it comes to eating, chew slowly, sit upright, and get relaxed. Be completely immersed in the action. Feel how your body—

your gut system—takes care of your food. In other words, tune in with your gut-brain connection.

- Keep a food diary. Dedicating a special journal for your 3-day gut cleanse is an excellent idea to keep track of the symptoms and changes that may occur during your reintroduction phase. But there's more. Starting this journey with a diary is a way to follow through the different processes and rules you should follow. Besides, it's the best way to jot down ideas and inspirations for meals and new insights you will learn along the way. So, a food diary is your best ally to make this journey personal and successful.

Key Foods

In this last step, you can add low-fiber food to your diet. Examples include white rice, pasta, eggs, tofu, ham, and bacon. Eating a small portion of baked goods is okay. For now, avoid highly processed food such as pizza, potato chips, and fast food. Also, make sure that your body is getting enough sources of probiotics in your main meal plan. You can still get some inspiration from the previous meal plans. Don't forget to take care of your brain-gut connection by getting enough sleep and doing some exercises. In this reintroduction phase, the key is to take the time to eat slowly and mindfully.

A Sample Meal Plan for Day 3

For breakfast, you can choose from the three alternatives below.

- Option 1: Banana, cornflakes with milk. This breakfast is super simple, yet, it is perfect for introducing new foods into your diet.
- Option 2: White toast, creamy peanut butter, and Greek Yogurt. Probiotics such as Greek yogurt are the best choice for a healthier gut.
- Option 3: Scrambled eggs and fruit juice. Eggs are a high-quality source of protein. This is definitely the best choice to have some protein intake in your breakfast.

For lunch, feel free to get inspired by the following options.

- Option 1: A tuna salad sandwich. To make this sandwich healthier, don't hesitate to add some veggies, such as celery, and don't forget to add lemon juice and garlic for seasoning.
- Option 2: Beef tacos with veggies. This lunch will make you feel full as it is filled with veggies

such as carrots and zucchini. For healthier and lower-calorie tacos, use olive oil and opt for lean ground beef.

- Option 3: Chicken and veggies soup with pasta soup. You can boil the pasta in a chicken broth and add some salt and fish sauce to make this soup tastier.

For dinner, you can choose between these options.

- Option 1: Baked salmon and white rice. Salmon is a super healthy food rich in omega-3. You can serve your dinner with some veggies if you want to. Though white rice is less nutritious than brown rice, it contains B vitamins and iron.
- Option 2: Pasta with olive oil and Parmesan cheese. The best way to cook pasta is to add some salt to the cooking water. If you want an easy dinner, this one's for you.
- Option 3: Tender roast beef cooked with cooked carrots. To obtain tender roast beef, use low temperatures for a long period of time.

Post-Cleanse Maintenance

- Drink plenty of water. Water is essential for diet, especially for digestion. When your body gets enough water, it facilitates digestion. It also helps to remove waste and toxins from your body. After the reintroduction phase, water plays a key part in helping the gut for digesting new food. Besides, it makes it easy for the body to adapt itself. In fact, it aids in breaking down the food you eat. So, when you reintroduce non-gut-friendly food, water is your best ally to support your digestion.

- Practice exercises. A lack of physical activities can cause digestive disorders such as constipation and bloating. Frequently exercising can help prevent those problems and improve gut health. As a matter of fact, researchers have found that exercise is beneficial for the gut microbiome. Daily exercises assist the gut in absorbing nutrients and make digestion easy and functional.

- Sleep. There is a correlation between sleep and the immune system. Sleep deprivation results in inflammation as the immune system produces excessive pro-inflammatory *cytokines*, an element responsible for inflammation

(Simpson, 2020). Moreover, when the body lacks sleep, it tends to crave more sugar. This is due to the hormone imbalance caused by sleep deprivation. Finally, when sleep isn't enough, you may become vulnerable to stress, which affects the gut microbiome through the gut-brain connection.

- Limit sugar intake. Artificial and refined sugar causes disturbance in the gut microbiome. It is harmful to the good bacteria in the gut system. As you try to reintroduce new food after the process, make sure to limit your sugar intake. You can do so by avoiding highly processed, sugary food. Be wary of soda and other sugary drinks as well. In your meal plan, be moderate when using sugar.

It is possible! It is possible and feasible to improve your well-being by shifting to a gut-friendly diet. Besides, you now have everything you need to know to practice the R.E.S.T.O.R.E method and successfully restore your gut health and achieve better well-being. And you have the goal to lose weight and get in better shape. This gut-cleanse journey will greatly help you to remove toxins, fats, and harmful elements from your digestive health. In fact, a super healthy body equals a thriving gut system. Not only is this method effective in inserting the right food into your diet, but it is also the best way to switch to a better lifestyle. As a matter of fact, you can consider this program as the door to change your entire well-being. Besides, a 3-day program is totally realistic, quite short, yet extremely efficient to prove to yourself that you can do it! As a matter of fact, you can eliminate inflammation, digestive problems, and chronic diseases one step at a time. You now hold the key to feeling healthy and great in your own skin.

As you've seen, food is crucial to repair and nurturing a healthier gut. Keep the key foods within your reach to help you in your shopping and make better food choices when ordering at the restaurant. Keep in mind that you can be a lot more creative (in fact, you are) and mix ingredients that are both tasty and beneficial for your gut. It will make your gut-friendly lifestyle more fun as well. And if a 3-day gut cleanse seems daunting to you, for now, don't worry! Know that you can always try to make it step by step by adding key foods to your diet. Thanks to the power of detoxifying foods, you are on the right path to creating a sustainable, healthier lifestyle. When it comes to food supplements, being aware of what's good and bad for your well-being is important. What's more, it's safe to understand the effects of detoxifying foods for your body so that you can make the best decisions to opt for the right supplements for yourself. If you are a complete beginner in the use of probiotics and prebiotics supplements, don't worry; natural foods are also great sources of nutrients and are packed with fiber, vitamins, and minerals. So, get ready because you're going to learn a lot of valuable information to live a better lifestyle, as you will no longer be unfamiliar with what's good for your gut and your overall well-being.

STEP 2: DETOXIFYING FOODS AND SUPPLEMENTING

4

SUPERFOODS FOR A SUPER GUT

Toxins are damaging to the digestive system and overall health. Elements such as pesticides, triclosan, arsenic, and BPA are present in the different materials and food you consume every day. However, these often go unnoticed as they are already included as components of the things you may use. Let's take the example of *triclosan* which can be found in mouthwash, toothpaste, and other self-care products. *Triclosan* is dangerous because it alters the gut microbes and changes the types of microbes living in the gut system (Lavage Wellness, 2017). What's more, it can bring about allergic diseases such as allergies and eczema. Another type of toxin used in different products is a pesticide. Not only does it kill insects, but it can also destroy the good bacteria present in your gastrointestinal tract. Yet, without the help of good bacteria, the body becomes vulnerable to chronic health diseases related to the gut and immune systems. Apart from that, soil and drinking water, being exposed to industrial pollution, may contain heavy metals such as cadmium, lead, and arsenic (Lavage Wellness, 2017). These can cause inflammatory diseases as they weaken the gut microbiome. Consequently, you must be aware of the presence of toxins in the food and products you use each day. Frequent exposure to toxins leads to disrupting the gut microbiome, altering the function of gut microbes, and causing serious health conditions.

Fortunately, food can save you. With the power of detoxifying foods, cleansing your gut from the effects of toxins is now possible and feasible regardless of your health goals and your diet. Most importantly, you can achieve great insights into the power of food to amplify your gut health and foster your well-being along the way. Natural foods are sources of power for the gut. The more you include detoxifying foods in your diet, the more you reduce the effects of toxins in your organism. In fact, some cleansing foods are extremely powerful to combat and eliminate toxins from your body. Besides, they are completely easy to find, and preparation doesn't take time and much effort.

DETOXIFYING FOODS FOR A HEALTHY GUT

Detoxifying Foods and Their Potential Benefits for Gut Health

When it comes to detoxification, one of the most important types of food you need to add to your diet is antioxidants. Did you know that antioxidants can prevent your cells from the damage of molecules called free radicals? Free radicals are dangerous for your cells as they are sources of illnesses and aging (Villines, 2017). They can be found in cigarette smoke, pollution, drugs, and pesticides. Cancer, autoimmune diseases, aging skin, heart, and cardiovascular diseases are the results of free radicals. Moreover, free radicals can cause oxidative stress causing damage to organs and tissues (Villines, 2017). Taking antioxidants in your diet helps to reduce the effects of these unstable molecules in your cells. The most-known antioxidant foods are asparagus, avocado, and beets.

Other important detoxifying foods are prebiotics which can be found in high-fiber foods. Dietary fiber is beneficial for the gut as it maintains the growth of the gut microbiome. How does it work exactly? So, dietary fiber fosters detoxifying enzymes in the liver and supports the liver from pro-inflammatory bacteria (Zoppi, 2021). What's more, it can effectively reduce the level of bad cholesterol in the organism. The most important sources of prebiotics are kidney beans, pinto beans, black beans, and lentils. But it can also be found in other vegetables such as beets, artichokes, red cabbages, sweet potatoes, broccoli, carrots, avocado, radishes, squash, pumpkins, kale, and spinach. Fruits such as berries, currants, and grapes are also great sources of prebiotics. Furthermore, there are detoxing herbs such as nori and coriander, which can destroy neurotoxins from the body. Finally, there are detoxification components in smoothies, green tea, and white tea.

A List of Detoxifying Foods and Their Specific Benefits for the Gut

Below is the list of the *most* detoxifying foods and the potential benefits they offer for your gut:

- Green veggies: Spinach, artichoke, kale, and broccoli are some excellent sources of magnesium that help to regulate the gut nerves. They contain an important antioxidant called *chlorophyll*, which aids in combating free radicals and supports the detoxification process (Wellbeingnutrition, 2023).
- Oats and apples: As soluble fibers, they facilitate bowels and help to regulate the rate of

gut motility. It's also a good idea to eat apples to reduce your appetite and get your fiber intake each day.

- Avocado and kale: Excellent antioxidants, they help to restore the cells of the gut. Avocado oil is one of the best foods for digestive health.
- Aloe vera: Containing antioxidants, aloe vera can calm the gut and improve the lining of the cells.
- Ginger: It is a great detox food as it enhances digestion, circulation, and sweating. It also helps to regulate the rate of gut motility and remove waste and toxins in the colon and liver (Wellbeingnutrition, 2023).
- Fermented food: Kefir, sauerkraut, and kombucha are part of fermented foods. They are helpful sources of probiotics for the gut microbiome. These are among the key foods you need to include in your diet if you want to replenish your gut after the elimination phase.
- Seasonal fruits: Are healthy sources of fibers. Seasonal fruits contribute to improving the gut flora and facilitating the bowels. They are also rich in nutrients, vitamins, and minerals. They don't take too much time to prepare. If you want to start adding fiber to your diet, fruits

can be your best option. Just make sure they are fresh and varied each day.

- Coconut oil: A powerful anti-bacterial, coconut oil also improves the absorption of nutrition. You can use it in your diet as it will add a different taste to your meals.
- Lemon: It improves digestion by helping the digestive system process food. Besides, it helps to reduce inflammation (Wellbeingnutrition, 2023). Lemon is perfect to season your food and gives a lighter taste to your meals.
- Flax and chia seeds. They contain fats and fiber that make it easy to digest food and get rid of waste, toxins, and cholesterol.
- Bone broth: Rich in protein and minerals, it is a gut-friendly food that promotes digestion and the intestinal lining.
- Garlic: It supports the gut in feeling the good bacteria in the gut system. It is rich in selenium and allicin, which are excellent detox components (Wellbeingnutrition, 2023).

Meal Ideas Featuring Detoxifying Foods for a Healthy Gut

For breakfast, you can opt for a green smoothie which is a great combination of spinach with mixed pineapple and bananas. It is super easy to do as you just mix all these ingredients to obtain a fresh and creamy smoothie. This breakfast is rich in fiber and potassium, and spinach is an excellent source of antioxidants.

For snacks, a fruit salad is perfect for getting a good dose of fiber and helps to give a sensation of fullness. How to choose the right fruits? Focus on seasonal fruits and make them as colorful as possible. In other words, the more variety you have in your fruit salad, the healthier it is. Don't hesitate to add probiotics fruits such as grapes or berries.

For lunch, a detox salad is an occasion to add green veggies and antioxidant sources to your diet. The food blog *Gimme Some Oven* suggests a combination of kale leaves, broccoli, red cabbage, and carrots for a super delicious salad detox (Gimme Some Oven, 2017). For your salad dressing, you can use olive oil, rice wine vinegar, black pepper, honey, and finely chopped ginger.

For dinner, a coconut lentil soup with lemongrass and ginger is a 100% detox recipe. You can cook the red lentils in the vegetable broth for about 20 minutes. Then, you can add coconut milk, ginger, garlic, and season with salt. It can be served with cooked rice if you want to.

THE ROLES OF VITAMINS AND SUPPLEMENTS IN DETOXIFYING THE GUT

Supplements are necessary for your detox journey to make sure that your body receives the proper amount of nutrients. Fortunately, natural foods are rich in nutrients. As you adopt the suggested meal plans in this book, you can be sure to have the right nutrient intake for yourself. Most importantly, supplements can help you balance your weight. To detox your body, antioxidants such as Vitamin C and E are powerful supplements to help you remove fats and toxins. For example, avocados, kiwifruit, and blackberries are healthier sources of these vitamins. Iron and Riboflavin can also assist in detoxing the liver (Palmer Lake Recovery, 2023). These are mostly found in nuts, wholemeal bread, dried fruits, legumes such as lentils, and dark leafy greens such as spinach and broccoli. What's more, Vitamin D, which you can fuel from exposure to sunlight, assists antioxidant genes and promotes immune functioning (Palmer Lake Recovery, 2023). Another important supplement you should consider is magnesium. It contributes to the detoxification phase and ensures metabolic functions (Palmer Lake Recovery, 2023). The most important sources of magnesium are spinach, chia seeds, almonds, soymilk, and peanuts.

Finally, there are probiotics that help to reduce oxidative stress and protect the intestinal barriers from toxins. Fermented foods and fermented vegetables are rich in probiotics. Examples include kefir, yogurt, cottage cheese, and sauerkraut.

The Importance of a Balanced Diet and Supplementing With Vitamins When Necessary

Above all, detoxification is a path to better health. Ensuring that your body gets enough nutrients is not an option. It's extremely important for your well-being. To prevent inflammation and other diseases, you need to adopt a balanced diet by varying your food and by being mindful of your body's needs. Supplements can be helpful only when there is an incapacity to get key foods. In fact, natural supplements are the best food for any type of diet, regardless of your health goals. They are sustainable and aren't cost-effective. When it comes to detoxification, preparing your food at home can help you monitor your meal plan and your nutrient intake. Therefore, strive to shop for fresh foods and focus on buying healthy and detoxifying foods.

A List of Vitamins and Supplements That Support Gut Health and Detoxification (Iliades, 2015)

- Vitamin D is essential for bone health as it helps to reduce bone and back pain. It also reduces the risk of colon cancer. It can be found in fatty fish, egg yolks, milk, juice, and cereal. Most importantly, you can fuel Vitamin D for your body through exposure to sunlight for a duration of 15 minutes.
- Magnesium is excellent for bone health and energy production. It also promotes sleep.
- Calcium is a fortifying nutrient. Sources of calcium are cereals, milk, cheese, yogurt, salty fish, broccoli and kale, nuts and nut butter, beans, and lentils.
- Zinc is helpful in boosting the immune system. It assists the body in using protein and fat for energy. Meat, seeds, dairy, whole grains, legumes, and eggs contain a high amount of zinc.
- Iron is a great source of energy. It promotes brain function as well and revitalizes the red blood cells. Iron is an essential mineral for the body and supports the creation of hemoglobin which brings oxygen from the lungs to all parts of the body.

- Vitamin B supports digestive systems. It can be found in fish, poultry, meat, and dairy products, as well as leafy greens and beans.
- Vitamin C is known as an antioxidant. It has multiple benefits for the immune system and digestion. Citrus fruits, berries, tomatoes, peppers, broccoli, and fortified cereal are sources of vitamin C.
- Vitamin A helps to strengthen the immune system, bone, and reproductive health. It can be found in leafy green vegetables such as kale and spinach, in orange and yellow vegetables such as carrots and sweet potatoes, and in other foods such as eggs, milk, red bell pepper, beef liver, and fish oils.

Can you believe that the food you eat each day is helpful in ensuring your well-being and achieving your health goals? Whether you aim to lose weight, balance your diet, or amplify your gut system, you can choose the right dietary supplements. What's unbelievable is the different nutrients, vitamins, and minerals that your body needs can be found in simple foods such as legumes, fruits, and vegetables. Moreover, you can change your diet by adding a new source of nutrients to each of your meals. However, keep in mind that when it comes to food and diet, balance is key. You must be moderate in your food supplement intake. To do so, strive to vary your meal whenever possible. Make sure that you are eating the right detoxifying foods that are essential for your health. Having a variety of nutrients will prevent you from getting health problems while helping your body to get stronger and healthier. In the next chapter, you will learn more about the use of probiotics and prebiotics in your diet. This is the most important part of this step because it will give you some ideas about natural food supplements as well as the different recommendations and advice when it comes to taking synthetic and artificial supplements.

5

THE GOOD BACTERIA STORY

The role of microbes in the gastrointestinal system has always been recognized in traditional food and modern lifestyle (Bagchi, 2014). They have been proven to be efficient for gut balance and reduce the effects of bad microbes. For that reason, the variety of fermented food in Western and Eastern gastronomies were born. For example, kefir is an Eastern Europe fermented drink produced from different milks such as goat, buffalo, sheep, camel, and cow. It contains a high number of good bacteria, essential for the gut. Another well-known fermented food is tempeh, which originated in Indonesia (Bagchi, 2014). It has been consumed for over 300 years and is also rich in protein and vitamins. So, not only are ferments rich in probiotics, but they also provide essential nutrients for the body.

WHAT ARE PROBIOTICS?

Probiotics are good bacteria living in the gut system and which are mostly found in fermented foods. These microbes ensure a key role in the function of the gastrointestinal tract. To be considered lively bacteria, they must be "isolated from a human and survive in the intestine after ingestion" (Cleveland Clinic, 2020). They mainly help the body restore the health of microorganisms in the gut and support the body's immune response. To gain all its benefits, they need to contain lively bacteria and be stored in a safe place with the right conditions.

How Do They Work

Probiotics ensure the good function of your gut. They strengthen your digestive health by eliminating harmful bacteria while revitalizing the immune system and intestinal motility (Cleveland Clinic, 2020). In other words, they contribute to maintaining the gut function by balancing good and bad bacteria. Hence, probiotics protect your gut from inflammation and diseases. They are mostly found in the large intestines. In your daily life, probiotics support your digestion, break down vitamins and medications, and strengthen your lining cells to prevent bad bacteria from accessing your blood (Cleveland Clinic, 2020). They also help to restore the bacteria destroyed by antibiotics.

Types of Probiotics

There are three types of probiotics. Firstly, there is *Lactobacillus* (Felson, 2017). It is the most known type of probiotic and can be found in yogurt and other fermented foods. Its role is to minimize inflammation, such as diarrhea, and assist in the digestion of lactose, the sugar in milk. Yogurt, sauerkraut, kefir, and sourdough bread are great sources of *Lactobacillus*. Secondly, there is *Bifidobacterium* which can be found in fermented foods that are rich in lactic acid bacteria (Felson, 2017). Examples include cultured milk and probiotic yogurt. It helps to alleviate the symptoms of irritable bowel syndrome. The third type of probiotic is *Saccharomyces boulardii*. It is a yeast found in probiotics and helps to defuse diarrhea and other digestive problems (Felson, 2017). Lychee, kombucha, and kefir all contain this type of bacteria. It's important to mention that all of these probiotics can be consumed in food, drinks, or in the form of capsules, pills, and powders.

What Do They Do

Probiotics play a major role in overall health: It maintains gut function by balancing the good and bad bacteria. It's important to note that the overgrowth of bad bacteria leads to diseases, while the diversity of good bacteria is a way to prevent diseases and keep the functionality of the digestive system. Probiotics ensure different functions by supporting digestion and protecting your body from bad bacteria. To do so, probiotics enhance the cells to combat toxins and prevent them from accessing the blood (Cleveland Clinic, 2020). They also help to absorb vitamins, nutrients, and medications. Besides, they can reduce the risk of cancer, improve oral health, and prevent allergies.

Benefits

Probiotics offer several benefits for the gut and overall well-being. By helping in the treatment of IBS, they are an excellent ally for the digestive system. They can prevent infectious diarrhea caused by viruses, bacteria, or parasites (Cleveland Clinic, 2020). What's more, they improve skin conditions and help fight allergies, colds, and skin problems such as eczema. Probiotics are also proven to have positive effects on the urinary and vaginal health.

What Probiotics Are Super Healthy?

The best probiotics are the ones found in fermented foods and drinks such as yogurt, pickles, kombucha, and kefir. With the variety of probiotics sources, you can create a healthy diet while getting the right amount of probiotics intake to support your gut system. For example, yogurt, sourdough bread, and buttermilk are great for breakfast. Cottage cheese, kombucha, and tempeh are perfect for lunch. Fermented sauerkraut, kimchi, and miso are excellent for dinner.

How to Use Them Safely?

To ensure the quality and efficiency of probiotics, they should be sheltered from heat, oxygen, light, and humidity (Felson, 2017). Such a condition needs to be respected to keep its benefits. Otherwise, they might die or break down. The surest way to keep them safe is by storing them in the refrigerator. Most importantly, when buying your probiotics, make sure you always check the labels and the expiration date, and follow the instructions properly.

Some people should be cautious before taking probiotics as they might endanger or worsen their health conditions. Examples include those who have a weakened immune system, such as those who have undergone chemotherapy. There are also risks of infection for people who had recent surgeries and critical illnesses.

When you decide to take probiotics, the following tips can be helpful for you before purchasing them.

- Choose the right type of probiotics according to your health conditions. Be sure to listen to professional advice before deciding. In fact, it's a good idea to have an assessment of your health conditions before taking any probiotics supplements, as certain types of probiotics can work for you for certain diseases while others can't. Besides, the two types of probiotics may not be combinable as well.
- Make it a habit to check the label. Make sure to read the components and the different ingredients, as well as the expiration date. Be aware of the different health conditions that are suitable for this specific type of probiotics. What's more, be cautious about the conditions for storage. Pay attention to the duration of the probiotics intake and the risks it may induce.
- Seek healthcare advice. Whether it's about choosing the type of probiotics or the amount you should take, it's always useful to elicit professional advice before adding probiotics supplements to your diet.

WHAT ARE PREBIOTICS?

Prebiotics are undigested food ingredients and serve as food sources for the bacteria living in the gut microbiota. They are mostly found in dietary fiber and contribute to the growth of probiotics. They also ensure different functions for the gut system. In fact, they fuel energy for your colon and assist in mucus production (Davani-Davari et al., 2019). To be considered as prebiotics, they go through different stages. For example, they shouldn't be digested by the gastrointestinal tract and must be "resistant to acid pH of the stomach" (Davani-Davari et al., 2019).

How Do They Work

Prebiotics can be dietary fibers or supplements. To survive, they pass through your digestive system and make their way to the colon, where they are fermented by microorganisms. This process is beneficial for your gut health as once they are absorbed by the organism through the fermentation process. They help to fight inflammation and support immunity.

Types of Prebiotics

Different types of prebiotics can be found in food and supplements. First, there are fructans, in which you can find *inulin* and *fructooligosaccharides* (Davani-Davari et al., 2019). Many vegetables contain inulin, such as asparagus, garlic, leeks, onions, and soybeans. Inulin is the prebiotic element that gives you the feeling of fullness after eating. What's more, it plays an important role in bowel movements. Another advantage of inulin is its power to reduce bad cholesterol, regulate blood sugars, and most importantly, preserve good bacteria in the gut. Inulin can be taken as supplements in the form of tablets, capsules, and powders. However, natural foods offer extra benefits in terms of nutrients as they are also rich in antioxidants and vitamins. Another type of prebiotic is resistant starches. Resistant to digestion, they are sources of food for the gut microbes in the colon. That's why they are essential for the maintenance of probiotics and for gut health. Green bananas, barley, oats, rice, beans, and legumes are the main sources of resistant starches. Then there is pectin, which is present in many fruits including apples, apricots, peaches, and raspberries. It is also present in some vegetables including carrots, green beans, tomatoes, and potatoes. So, pectin is an excellent source of antioxidants and helps to improve the skin cells in the intestinal lining. It is beneficial for the gut system by promoting the diversity of microbes in the gut. Besides, it helps to defuse bacterial diseases.

How Are They Different From Probiotics?

Prebiotics are non-digestible high-fiber foods that are essential for the living microorganisms in the gut, whereas the probiotics contain the good bacteria living in the gut. Probiotics are responsible for the gut balance, and prebiotics help them in growth and diversity. They are interdependent and ensure the function of the gut system.

Benefits

Prebiotics provide multiple benefits for health. Firstly, they facilitate bowel movements. It means that consuming many high-fiber foods reduces constipation (Davani-Davari et al., 2019). Prebiotics enhance good bacteria called *bifidobacteria*, which is helpful for bowel movement. Secondly, prebiotics help to absorb minerals that your body needs. Examples include magnesium, calcium, and phosphorus. Most importantly, they boost the immune system and increase the body's natural defenses and immune function. Apart from that, eating prebiotic foods reduces the sensation of hunger and makes you feel full longer, which prevents cravings. As a matter of fact, the presence of oligofructose, a type of dietary fiber found in foods like onions, Jerusalem artichoke, leeks, and garlic, can reduce the hunger hormone ghrelin and suppresses appetite. There are other benefits of eating prebiotic foods. For instance, they help to regulate blood sugar and effectively lower bad cholesterol. What's more, they are powerful anti-inflammatory thanks to their production of good bacteria in the gut system. By maintaining the growth of gut microbiota, they lessen the risks of getting chronic diseases such as obesity, cardiovascular diseases, and diabetes (Cleveland Clinic, 2022). Hence, not only do prebiotics essential for the gut, but they are also beneficial for physical well-being.

What Prebiotics Are Super Healthy?

Garlic

Garlic is one of the best prebiotic foods thanks to its components and the benefits it offers. Research proves that garlic can minimize the risk of cardiovascular diseases and blood glucose levels. It is also an excellent antioxidant and anti-inflammatory. Garlic is one of the dietary fibers that helps to produce good bacteria, such as *bifidobacteria*, which helps to improve bowel movements (Cleveland Clinic, 2022).

Onions

Onions contain inulin, the type of prebiotic that has several benefits: Maintain the good bacteria in the gut, enhance the immune system, and improve bowel movements. It has antioxidant and anticancer properties as well, thanks to the existence of *flavonoid quercetin*

(Cleveland Clinic, 2022). Furthermore, onions are rich in antibiotics which are essential for the cardiovascular system.

Bananas

Bananas are rich in resistant starches, another type of prebiotics that strengthen gut bacteria as they resist digestion. Bananas also contain vitamins, minerals, and inulin.

Oats

Oats have multiple benefits. As resistant starch, they are important for the gut flora by helping the growth of beneficial bacteria. What's more, oats are proven to reduce the risk of cancer, regulate appetite, and reduce bad cholesterol.

Apples

Rich in antioxidants and fiber, apples are nutritious and an excellent ally for gut health. They contain pectin, which helps to nurture the cells in the intestinal lining. It is also perfect for a weight loss diet as it has low calories and reduces the feeling of hunger. Apart from that, apples are beneficial for digestion and can decrease the risk of diabetes, cancer, and heart disease.

Tips to Eating Prebiotics Safely

There's no downside to eating fruits and vegetables. However, you must be moderate, especially if you intend to change your diet and switch to a more fiber-rich one. Therefore, try to introduce new foods step by step and strive to vary your meal plan. Apart from that, avoid eating prebiotics late in the evening to prevent digestive problems as "microorganisms are less active during the night," which could induce indigestion (Cleveland Clinic, 2022). Eating a small portion of different fruits is a good idea to test how your body reacts to prebiotics. So, balance is the key when it comes to eating prebiotics. Also, make sure that you have enough fiber intake each day for healthier long-term benefits for your gut and your health.

CHOOSING THE RIGHT PROBIOTIC SUPPLEMENT

Foods and Beverages Versus Supplements

Strive to eat natural probiotic foods as they are always better than supplements and bring more other benefits for your body. In fact, they are less risky for your health and are combinable with any type of diet. Besides, they are easy to prepare and don't take too much of your time. So, prioritize natural food and drinks over supplements whenever possible.

What Supplements to Use

Choosing the right supplements is important. First, find out if eating supplements is suitable and safe for your health. Make sure that your health condition is favorable for probiotics supplements. In the case of health and immune system problems, it's safe to ask for healthcare advice before taking probiotics. Second, focus on quality. Don't hesitate to look for recommendations if you want to be sure about which brand to choose. Finally, prioritize high-quality ingredients without artificial additives or fillers.

Check the Strains

Bacteria have three names: genus, species, and strain. For example, in *Bifidobacterium longum W11*, *Bifidobacterium* is the genus, *longum* is the species, and *W11* is the strain (Moore, n.d.). To achieve the benefits of probiotics intake, these three must be complete and mentioned on the label.

CFU Count

Colony Forming Units or CFUs are the number of bacteria you can find in a supplement (Moore, n.d.). CFUs vary from one to 10 billion CFUs but should contain at least the genus *Lactobacillus, Bifidobacterium, Bacillus,* or *Saccharomyces boulardii.* If you don't have enough bacteria, you might not attain the desired effects. In this case, more is better, but it also depends on other factors, such as the type of treatment and your expected results.

Check Other Important Information on the Label

The storage condition, the ingredients, the expiration date, and the manufacturer are key information you should look for in a label. For storage, the fridge can be the best place to store probiotics, especially for heat-dried formulas, while freeze-dried ones can be kept at room temperature (Moore, n.d.). Regarding ingredients, check for allergies or any food intolerances and focus on those which contain inulin, an important food source for bacteria. Pay attention to the expiration date as well, as it affects the dose and the effects of CFUs.

Consider the Science and Clinical Studies

Be aware of the research and clinical studies that prove the efficiency and the quality of the probiotics you purchase. A brand supplement backed by research is always trustworthy and should be prioritized. Also, do your research about the brand name or ask for recommendations from professionals.

Does It Matter What Form of Probiotic You Choose?

The strain, the CFU count, and your health conditions are critical elements for choosing the best supplement for you. As most of them can treat IBS symptoms, the CFU and the strain vary from one supplement to another. Therefore, it's crucial to pick the one that is suitable for you. One brand supplement might be extremely efficient for one person but not for another, as it also depends on the treatments and the health conditions of each individual. Depending on the ingredients they contain, some supplements might have undesirable effects for vegans, lactose intolerance, and other allergies.

How to Tell if Probiotics Are High-Quality

CFU count and strain are key factors in determining the quality of a probiotics supplement. Another criterion is the third-party test as it is more trustworthy than the price itself though the price can justify the research and the tests realized to prove the quality of the supplement. In other words, read carefully to the label to find out if the probiotics are high quality.

Choosing Probiotics for Your Health Needs

When it comes to picking the right supplement, you should consider your health conditions and the type of treatment. Consider the duration of the treatment as well. The strain and CFU count are other decisive factors for getting effective results. Opting for the right supplement helps to avoid downside effects and allergies.

Two words that could sum up your gut health are probiotics and prebiotics. Whether you are familiar with your digestive system or not, these are the most important components of the gastrointestinal tract. Probiotics are considered as the microorganisms living in your gut, helping the digestive system to function properly. These can mostly be found in fermented dairy and vegetables. They offer multiple benefits for health in the treatment of IBS, allergies, and skin problems. Probiotics can be obtained from fermented foods or supplements. The best sources of probiotics are probiotic yogurt, kefir, sauerkraut, and tempeh. If you take probiotics supplements, make sure that you store them properly by following the indications on the label. It's important to note that people who have gone through serious treatments with weakened immune systems, such as chemotherapy, shouldn't avoid taking probiotics supplements. Prebiotics, on the other hand, are indigested food groups that are mostly found in fiber-rich food and supplements. Their main role is to maintain the growth of good bacteria in the gut. Prebiotics play different roles in the gastrointestinal tract by supporting bowel movements, defusing bacterial diseases, and enhancing the immune system. Prebiotics have anti-inflammatory properties as well. Natural foods are the best prebiotics sources as they provide vitamins and minerals for the body. When it comes to eating fiber-rich foods, you should be moderate and avoid taking them late at night to avoid the risk of indigestion. Supplements can be helpful to meet your daily prebiotics intake according to your treatment and circumstances. When taking food supplements, keep in mind that your health conditions and the types of treatments matter. In the next chapter, we'll go into detail about the power of digestive enzymes and dietary fiber to break down foods and strengthen digestion efficiently. Finally, you'll come to understand how fermented food works and which ones you should adopt in your diet.

"Health is the greatest of human blessings."

— HIPPOCRATES

We're beginning to hear more about the gut-brain connection and the importance of gut health for overall well-being... Yet there are still a shocking number of people living in a constant state of mild discomfort that they've become so accustomed to they barely notice anymore.

You're here reading this book because you knew you wanted to make a change. As you discover more and begin implementing the R.E.S.T.O.R.E method, you're going to feel a marked difference in both mind and body – and you'll probably wish you'd learned all of this far earlier.

You can't go back in time and give yourself the advice you wish you'd had then, but you *can* help someone else get there quicker.

Improving gut health has such a significant impact on our overall quality of life that I'm passionate about

getting this guidance out to as many people as I can –
and you can help me.

**By leaving a review of this book on Amazon, you'll
show other people where they can find all the information they need to overhaul their gut health and
improve their overall quality of life.**

Simply by telling new readers how this book has helped
you and what they'll find inside, you'll show them just
how important their gut health is and guide them
towards the path they need to take to improve it.

Thank you for your support. Many people are living
with both mental and physical discomfort that could
easily be avoided by making these simple changes, and
I'm determined to help as many of them as I can –
thank you for helping me to do that.

6

THE FIBER FIX

Fiber encompasses a variety of non-digestive plant foods such as carbohydrates, fruits, vegetables, and whole grains. Fiber foods are rich in nutrients, vitamins, and minerals. In addition to that, fiber is beneficial for the digestive system as it provides a source of nutrition for the gut microbes. It becomes prebiotics after fermentation in the colon. That's why it reinforces the gut flora and helps the microbes thrive in the gut. Fiber also ensures the regularity of bowel movements (Fields, 2010). In fact, the insoluble fiber becomes stool bulk which then contributes to removing waste and toxins from the body. It means that the more fiber you have in your diet, the easier it is for the body to expel them. Fiber is the best food to fight constipation and diarrhea and prevents inflammation.

Aside from its actions on digestive health, fiber is an excellent ally to control and lose weight. As a matter of fact, high-fiber foods provide a feeling of fullness and satiety, which prevents low-calorie intake (Fields, 2010). By consuming a large portion of fiber each day, you can control your hunger and avoid cravings. According to researchers, soluble fiber promotes the diversity of bacteria in the gut, which reduces the risk of belly fat. Soluble fiber sources include flaxseeds, sweet potatoes, apricots, oranges, and oatmeal. Most importantly, fiber foods contain low calories and are heart-healthy. It minimizes the risk of colon cancer and cardiovascular diseases.

DIGESTIVE ENZYMES

What Are Digestive Enzymes?

Digestive enzymes are substances the body produces to break down food and nutrients. The body creates these enzymes in the mouth, the pancreas, the stomach, and the small intestine (Pietrangelo, 2020). A lack of digestive enzymes can cause gastrointestinal symptoms, malnutrition, and poor digestion. They also ensure the absorption of nutrients for the body. In fact, with the role of digestive enzymes, the nutrients will only pass through the digestive system and go to waste.

How Do Digestive Enzymes Work in the Gut?

The digestive process starts from the moment you consume food. The digestive enzymes present in the mouth ensure your body can absorb the food. Then, the process continues until the nutrients are absorbed through the wall of the small intestine and disposed of through the bloodstream (Pietrangelo, 2020). The body releases digestive enzymes when you anticipate eating, smelling, and tasting food, and experience the digestive process. When it comes to replacement digestive enzymes, these should be taken before eating in order to ease digestion and process food easily.

Replacement digestive enzymes break down carbs, proteins, and fats if the pancreas doesn't produce natural enzymes (Pietrangelo, 2020). It's important to mention that the shortage of digestive enzymes is one of the causes of stomach aches, diarrhea, and gas.

Types of Digestive Enzymes

The main types of digestive enzymes are amylase, lipase, protease, maltase, and sucrase (Pietrangelo, 2020). Produced by the salivary glands and the pancreas, amylase is important to absorb carbohydrates or starches into sugar molecules. Lack of amylase may induce diarrhea, but excessive amylase in the blood can be a sign of pancreas injury, pancreas cancer, and pancreas inflammation. Another digestive enzyme is lipase which helps the liver bile to manage fats and turn them into fatty acids and glycerol. Lipase is secreted by the mouth, the stomach, and the pancreas. Shortage of this digestive enzyme leads to a lack of fat-soluble vitamins such as A, D, E, and K. Then, there are proteases that are produced by the stomach and the pancreas. They break down proteins into amino acids and prevent bacteria and yeasts from reaching the intestines. Lack of proteases can lead to allergy and toxicity in the intestines. Proteases ensure cell division, the blood clotting and reinforce immune function (Pietrangelo, 2020). Apart from that, both maltase and sucrase are secreted by the small intestine and promote the absorption of sugar. Maltase manages to turn maltose—malt sugar—into glucose, while sucrase—the sugar in table sugar—transforms sucrose into fructose and glucose (Pietrangelo, 2020).

Sources of Digestive Enzymes

The main sources of digestive enzymes are the salivary glands, stomach, pancreas, and small intestine (Pietrangelo, 2020). The salivary glands secrete amylase beforehand to break down carbs. Amylase is also produced by the pancreas to reinforce the digestion of carbs. Pancreas also secretes lipase to turn fats into fatty acids. Pancreas helps them in the production of digestive enzymes, although it doesn't have a specific role in digestion. The stomach also supplies the body with digestive enzymes by handling proteins. Lastly, the small intestine provides different digestive enzymes such as lactase, maltase, and sucrase to absorb sugar and moves it to the bloodstream and throughout the tissues.

Conditions That Affect Digestive Enzyme Production

Two important conditions can alter the secretion of enzymes. One of them is lactose intolerance. When the small intestine doesn't produce lactase—which transforms natural sugar in milk into lactose—it's impossible for the body to digest lactose in dairy products (Powell Key, 2021). Lactose intolerance can be genetic from birth or caused by circumstances such as illness, injury, and surgery. Exocrine pancreatic insufficiency, which manifests through pancreas inflammation, pancreatic cancer, and cystic fibrosis, can prevent the pancreas from secreting digestive enzymes as well. Fortunately, different foods can support the production of enzymes.

Food That Contains Natural Digestive Enzymes

Several natural foods are high in digestive enzymes. For instance, raw honey contains both amylase and protease (Powell Key, 2021). Eating honey promotes the absorption of carbohydrates and proteins. To support gut health, you can use it to sweeten your food or include it in yogurt. Other important sources of digestive enzymes are papaya and avocados. Papaya can supply your body with protease, while avocados can produce lipase. It's easy to add them to your diet to enjoy all the benefits they provide for your body. Apart from that, sauerkraut or fermented cabbage can create different digestive enzymes to break down protein, fats, and starches during the fermentation process.

Digestive Enzyme Supplementation

If natural foods are insufficient to help the production of digestive enzymes, pancreatic enzyme replacement, which is only available through prescription, can be helpful. In fact, this therapy can help in the treatment of chronic pancreatitis, pancreatic cancer, cystic fibrosis, diabetes, and even lactose intolerance, as research has proved that taking lactase enzyme before eating dairy can lessen lactose intolerance (Ianiro et al., 2016). It also aids in the treatment of digestive and malabsorption disorders. Digestive enzyme replacement is important for IBS symptoms such as diarrhea, constipation, and stomach pain. Enzyme supplements can be produced from animal sources or microbial sources. As a matter of fact, some of them may contain a diversity of digestive enzymes such as amylase, lipase, and protease.

Risks and Potential Side Effects of Digestive Enzyme Supplementation

Taking digestive enzyme supplements can disturb digestion and cause digestive disorders such as constipation, nausea, abdominal cramps, diarrhea, gas, bloating, loose stools or greasy stools, and stomach discomfort (Pietrangelo, 2020). Not taking the right dose or the ratio of enzymes might be the reason behind those undesirable effects. Hence, for your safety, it's crucial to ask for a doctor's advice to determine the right dosage and read the label carefully to check ingredients and food sensitivities before purchasing a supplement.

FIBER IN YOUR DIET

What Is Dietary Fiber?

Dietary fiber is the substance in plant foods that the body can't digest. It is a part of carbohydrate that is resistant to digestion, whereas most carbohydrates are transformed into glucose (Harvard School of Public

Health, 2018). Dietary fiber is super healthy and plays a major role in the gut microbiota. However, too much fiber intake can cause digestive problems, gas, and intestinal blockages (Aswell, 2018). Besides, eating a variety of fiber is more beneficial than eating the same fiber supplement, as the latter can damage the intestinal biome and the protective mucus wall.

Types of Fiber

There are two types of fiber: soluble fiber and insoluble fiber. Soluble fiber can be dissolved in water. It includes pectins, resistant starch, inulin, and Guar gum. Pectins are naturally found in apples and berries. They have laxative effects and contribute to regulating blood sugar and cholesterol levels. Resistant starch includes legumes, unripe bananas, cooked pasta, and potatoes. They add bulk to stool and don't have a laxative effect. Inulin can be found in onions, chicory root, asparagus, and Jerusalem artichokes. With a laxative effect, it helps to bulk stool and acts as a prebiotic. Guar gum is a "fermented fiber isolated from seeds" and is often used as a thickener for foods (Harvard School of Public Health, 2018). Insoluble fiber promotes stool bulk formation as it reduces constipation and irregular stools. Whole-wheat flour, nuts, beans and vegetables, cauliflower, green beans, and potatoes all contain insoluble fiber.

How Fiber Works in the Gut

Fiber goes through different stages in the gut. Insoluble fiber moves quickly through the stomach as it can't be absorbed by the digestive tract, whereas soluble fiber fills the stomach and gives a feeling of satiety and fullness (Aswell, 2018). The latter adds bulk to stools. Bacteria transform dietary fiber into short-chain fatty acids, which are then broken down by the body. Short-chain fatty acids stimulate the metabolic process and maintain the vitality of the colon (Aswell, 2018).

Natural Supplements for Fiber

Fruits and vegetables are the main sources of fiber though certain foods tend to have high amounts of fiber, such as beans, peas, celery, leafy greens, oatmeal, and lentils. Whole grains such as amaranth, pearl barley, wheat berries, quinoa, and whole wheat couscous are also one of the best dietary fibers. To diversify your diet, you can add chickpeas, split peas, apples, almonds, chia seeds, brussels sprouts, and avocado to your meal plans (Aswell, 2018). To boost your fiber intake, you can try eating fresh fruits and potatoes with their skin on. It is recommended to take 38 grams of fiber per day for men and 25 grams a day for women. To increase your fiber intake, start the day with a fiber-rich breakfast with whole grains cereals or oatmeal. By taking enough fiber each day, you reap the benefits of fiber. It can lower blood pressure and cholesterol level and helps to control your blood sugar, your weight, and your calorie intake. When it comes to digestive health, fiber ensures regular bowel movements and can minimize hemorrhoids and small pouches in the colon. To optimize your gut health, avoid taking refined foods as they are stripped of fiber. Examples include white bread and pasta. Finally, strive to eat seasonal fruits as they are fresher and add diversity to your fiber intake. For snacks, you can opt for fresh fruits, raw vegetables, and whole-grain crackers.

Benefits of Fiber Supplementation

Fiber supplements are mainly produced from soluble and insoluble fibers. Some of them contain inulin fiber and antioxidants from tea (Aswell, 2018). It is useful to mention that fiber supplements lack vitamins and minerals. However, if you struggle to meet your daily intake, fiber supplements can be helpful to reach the right amount. Research proved that fiber supplements could offer similar benefits to natural fiber sources (Griffin, n.d.). For example, taking supplements can help to decrease the risk of heart disease and lower the risk of diabetes. Soluble fiber has positive effects on controlling cholesterol levels, whereas insoluble fiber can regulate your stools. To boost your digestive health, you can combine fiber supplements with other nutrients such as zinc, collagen, and probiotics (Griffin, n.d.). Always consider your needs to purchase the right supplement. Some conditions that require a fiber supplement include constipation, cholesterol reduction, and blood sugar regulation, along with the duration of the treatment. Finally, you can consider other criteria, such as your budget.

Sources and Types of Fiber Supplementation

Fiber supplements are made from soluble and insoluble fibers. Some of them contain inulin fiber and antioxidants from tea. *Psyllium*, a type of fiber supplement, is produced from 70% of soluble fiber and 30% of insoluble fiber (Griffin, n.d.). It is fermented in the gut and becomes a nutritious food for good bacteria. Psyllium is effective for the treatment of constipation and IBS. Another type of fiber supplement is *Methylcellulose*. It is mainly created from the soluble fiber of the cell walls of plants. Non-allergic and non-fermentable fiber, Methylcellulose can help in regulating bowel movements and fighting constipation. Lastly, *Polycarbophil* is a soluble fiber that adds bulk to stools (Griffin, n.d.). It can be used to treat constipation and irregular bowel movements.

CONDITIONS THAT BENEFIT FROM FIBER SUPPLEMENTATION

Fiber supplements are used for the treatment of IBS, constipation, blood cholesterol, and blood sugar. They are helpful to stimulate and improve bowel movements as well. Weight-loss diet can also benefit from fiber supplements to manage appetite and reduce cravings.

Risks and Potential Side Effects of Fiber Supplementation

Common side effects of taking fiber supplements concern digestive disorders such as severe abdominal pain, gas, diarrhea, constipation, and bloating (Tresca, 2022). These are often due to the abrupt fiber intake your gut must experience. Interference with other medications can also induce undesirable effects on your health. The dosage can also affect your health conditions. Therefore, it's better to start with a small dose.

FERMENTED FOOD AND HOW IT BENEFITS YOUR GUT AND BODY

Fermented foods are a variety of foods and beverages that are processed through microbial growth with the transformation of ingredients through "enzymatic action". These are yogurt, kefir, cottage cheese, fermented vegetables, vegetable brine drinks, and kombucha tea. Fermentation has always been used for food preservation and flavoring. Fermented foods are excellent for gut health are they contain probiotics. According to researchers, they aid in reducing inflammation related to chronic diseases such as type 2 diabetes, rheumatoid arthritis, and chronic stress (Tresca, 2022). Less gut diversity means an increase of bad bacteria, one of the causes of inflammation. Fortunately, eating fermented foods promotes gut diversity thanks to the presence of good bacteria. What's more, it helps to prevent a leaky gut by strengthening the intestine wall. A leaky gut occurs when the intestine wall loses its permeability and becomes vulnerable to toxins. But fermented food is simply beneficial for digestive health by improving digestion and the immune system. The existence of lactic acid bacteria in fermented food reduces the risk of liver, breast, and intestine cancer as it prevents tumors from developing, according to some research (Wu et al., 2021). Moreover, eating fermented food positively affects the feel-good hormone called *serotonin*. It helps in finding sleep and alleviates anxiety and depression. Therefore, eating fermented foods such as yogurt, sauerkraut, and kimchi before bedtime can be helpful. However, it's important to mention that eating fermented food has side effects such as bloating and gas. This is due to the excess of gas after probiotics neutralize bad bacteria (Wu et al., 2021).

THE KIND OF FERMENTED FOODS THAT ARE HEALTHY

The fermentation process is successful when the bacteria absorb lactose or sugar with active cultures, which can produce a variety of healthy and concentrated probiotics foods such as kefir, plain yogurt, cottage cheese, gluten-free tempeh, refrigerated miso and sauerkraut, kimchi, and kombucha (Sanders, 2019). When choosing the right fermented food, pay attention to the label natural fermentation to ensure the ingredients contain live and active cultures.

NOT ALL FERMENTED FOODS ARE EQUAL

Kefir

Produced from a mixture of kefir grains—a combination of yeast and bacteria—and milk, kefir is a cultured dairy product that tastes like a thicker yogurt (Ajmera, 2020). It contains less amount of lactose than milk and can be consumed with smoothies and milk. Kefir is high in probiotics and antioxidants. Like any fermented food, kefir is excellent for digestive health and prevents inflammation.

Kombucha

Produced from green and black tea, kombucha is a fermented drink that provides health benefits. In fact, it helps to protect the liver from harmful chemicals and lower bad cholesterol and blood sugar (Ajmera, 2020).

Sauerkraut

Sauerkraut is a fermented cabbage that is low in calories and rich in fiber and vitamins. It can be served as casseroles, soups, or sandwiches. Unpasteurized sauerkraut is the best option to choose if you want to increase your probiotics intake.

Miso

Miso is a Japanese seasoning based on fermented soybeans with salt and koji, a type of fungus (Ajmera, 2020). It is often served with miso soup for breakfast and with cooked vegetables, or as a flavor for salad dressings, marinated meat, and salmon. Apart from its benefits on digestive health, miso is a heart-healthy food as well.

Natto

Natto is a traditional Japanese cuisine made from fermented soybeans. Eating natto can improve your digestive health by regulating your bowel movements and adding bulk to your stools (Ajmera, 2020). It is also a remedy for constipation. Besides, it is rich in vitamin K, which ensures calcium metabolism and strengthens bone health. The existence of natto helps to balance blood pressure and eliminate blood clots.

Tempeh

Made from the fermentation of soybeans, tempeh is concentrated in probiotics. Not only is it gut-friendly food, but it is also excellent for the heart by preventing chronic and cardiovascular diseases. For your diet, tempeh can be baked, steamed, and sauteed.

Kimchi

Originating from Korea, Kimchi is a type of fermented food produced from cabbages and radishes (Ajmera, 2020). Eating kimchi aids in reducing bad cholesterol and insulin resistance—a high level of insulin equals high blood sugar and insulin resistance.

Probiotic Yogurt

Probiotic yogurt is made from fermented milk. It is concentrated in calcium, potassium, phosphorus, riboflavin, and vitamin B12 (Ajmera, 2020). To optimize your health, it's better to opt for yogurt with live cultures and less sugar, for example, a plain non-fat Greek yogurt. For a balanced weight and blood pressure, you can sweeten yogurt with honey, fruits, or peanut butter.

A healthy gut goes hand in hand with good digestion. To help the body in absorbing foods, digestive enzymes are essential. As a matter of fact, they process food all through the gastrointestinal tract. Enzymes are created the moment you think about eating. That's why, eating enzyme supplements is beneficial for enzyme secretion and supports digestion. Natural enzymes are secreted by the mouth, the pancreas, the stomach, and the small intestine. Each type of enzyme plays a role in the digestive process. Natural enzyme sources are raw honey, papaya, avocado, and certain fermented foods such as sauerkraut. To ensure that your body expels toxins and waste, eating dietary fiber is crucial to regulate bowel movements. Regardless of your diet and your health goals, you need to evacuate waste and toxins for your overall well-being. Therefore, you should always have dietary fiber in your diet, especially fiber-rich foods such as leafy greens, whole grains, legumes, and fruits. You can also take fiber supplementation to meet your daily fiber intake, although supplements are devoid of minerals and vitamins. Lastly, fermented foods are super healthy for your gut as they contain probiotics. You can have them as a supplement in your meal to support your digestive system. Now that we've uncovered the essential foods for your gut, we'll dive deep into the gut-brain-muscle connection and discover the secrets to minimizing stress and optimizing your gut health through specific exercises, yoga poses, and meditations.

STEP 3: GENTLE EXERCISE AND STRESS REDUCTION

7

THE GUT-BRAIN-MUSCLE CONNECTION

THE ROLE OF EXERCISE IN GUT HEALTH

Exercise is, above all, a healthy lifestyle to gain strength and vitality. It is the best way to control your weight and get rid of toxins. In addition to that, it helps to distribute oxygen and blood flow throughout the body (Chai, n.d.). Interestingly, a healthier gut is proven to improve performance in physical activities, but what about the effects of exercise on gut health? According to researchers, physical activities practiced regularly can stimulate the gut microbiome and increase the production of short-chain fatty acids (Chai, n.d.). The latter aids in fighting inflammation and balancing blood sugar. Some types of exercises are highly recommended for gut health, such as aerobics, jogging, cycling, rowing, swimming, and skipping. So, exercise is effective in one condition: practiced with consistency and regularity. To improve gut health through exercise, nutrition is crucial. Other conditions include going outdoors for immersion in the natural environment. But when it comes to physical activities, starting small is the key to achieving long-term benefits.

How Exercise Impacts Gut Motility

Age, genetics, meditations, lifestyle, diet, stress, and antibiotics intake can influence the gut. However, other important factors, such as exercising, shouldn't be neglected. In fact, the practice of sports and physical activities contributes to the diversity of gut microbiome. The more diverse the gut microbiota, the more it produces short-chain fatty acids (Chai, n.d.). Having a healthier gut reduces the risk of chronic diseases, eases digestion, and positively impacts gut motility. In fact, exercising promotes the production of Vitamin B and K, which are important for the digestive process. Besides, daily exercises are proven to increase the production of anti-inflammatory molecules and decrease the bacteria associated with obesity and irritable bowel syndrome. In other words, exercising is advantageous to optimize gut health and maintain a balanced weight.

Benefits of a Diverse and Robust Gut Microbiome

A diverse and vital gut microbiome is beneficial for many reasons. As we've seen earlier, a healthy gut equals less risk of inflammation thanks to the production of short-chain fatty acids by probiotics. But what about the advantages of a diverse gut microbiome daily? First, a healthy gut ensures good digestion. It provides a feeling of ease and comfort for the body. It relieves pain and discomfort that comes with bad digestion: bloating, constipation, gas, etc. Second, a strong gut microbiome plays a key role in breaking down nutrients. It is vain to eat nutritious food if the gut cannot break it down. The gut ensures the nutrition is absorbed by the body and distributed through the bloodstream. Third, a healthy digestive tract helps to remove waste from the body. The fact that the body can get rid of waste through bowel movements in a regular way is the function of a healthy gut. Other advantages include the role of the gut in metabolic function and the immune system (Chai, n.d.). Let's not forget that a strong and diverse gut microbiome amplifies intestinal permeability and prevents leaky gut as well.

Exercise's Role in Reducing Inflammation in the Gut

The practice of daily exercises is the key to enhancing the gut-brain-muscle connection. Exercising alleviates stress and gets your mind off emotional strains. When your mind gets relaxed, it affects your gut in a positive way, as stress can cause disturbance to digestion in different ways: nausea, constipation, diarrhea, and so forth. Indeed, when you choose to release stress by doing exercises, you influence your gut system. Consequently, a strong gut impacts the gut composition by the increase of good bacteria and the decrease of bad bacteria. Yet, inflammation takes place when there are fewer good bacteria and more bad bacteria. Hence, daily exercises can minimize inflammation. However, a healthy gut goes hand in hand with a balanced lifestyle. It encompasses an enriched and gut-friendly diet, the practice of stress relief such as meditation, and of course, regular exercises. Such a lifestyle aids in reducing IBS and IBC as well. What's more, regular exercises can improve bowel movements and influence the secretion of digestive enzymes in the case of constipation. Exercise=bowel movements and digestive enzymes in the case of constipation

Types of Exercise for Optimal Gut Health

Sit-Ups

Sit-ups can effectively improve gut health by reducing bloating. You can practice it by lying on the floor, crossing your arms over your chest, and trying to lift your back by engaging your ab muscles. Then, get back to your initial position by still relying on your ab muscles. To get positive results, it's better to practice five times a week with eight to 10 repetitions per session.

Yoga

Yoga is the perfect exercise to optimize the gut-brain-muscle connection as it helps to reduce stress and lessen indigestion and IBS. Best gut-friendly yoga poses include triangle, downward dog, upward dog, boat, and child's pose (Allied Digestive Health, 2022). In fact, the practice of yoga affects the muscles by increasing center strength which is crucial for gut health. We'll explain more about these poses later on in this chapter.

Brisk Walking

Daily walking is a simple exercise that is beneficial for the gut system. As a matter of fact, walking stimulates the gastrointestinal system, enhances the digestive system, and helps in removing waste (Allied Digestive Health, 2022). With regular walking, you can benefit from normal defecation and reduced gas and swelling. The key is to practice walking 20 to 30 minutes a day, three to five times a week.

Pelvic Floor Exercises

To practice pelvic floor exercises, this is how you do it: Make yourself comfortable by taking a sitting position and squeezing your pelvic floor muscles 10 to 15 times. Keep each squeeze for a few seconds, and always breathe in a normal way. This exercise which restores the pelvic muscles, can help in defecation and bladder control (Allied Digestive Health, 2022).

Deep Breathing

Breathing exercises have tremendous benefits for health. For example, they can help in controlling your heart rate, release muscle tension, and increase blood oxygenation. Deep breathing exercises also aid in lowering your blood pressure. Besides, practicing regular deep breathing can get you relaxed as it helps to lessen stress hormones. What about gut health? Doing some breathing exercises before a meal contributes to improving digestion as it facilitates the secretion of digestive enzymes (Manaker, 2021). Keep in mind that hydration, yoga, exercises, and sleep can also influence digestion in a positive way. For those with gastroin-testinal symptoms, deep breathing helps in massaging the abdominal organs. To start, take a comfortable position by sitting or lying. Next, put your left hand on your chest and your right one on your belly. Then, take a deep breath through your nose for about four seconds and enjoy the feeling of your abdomen expanding. Try to hold your breath for two seconds. Afterward, exhale slowly through your mouth for six seconds. You can repeat the same exercise for five to 15 minutes.

Leg Elevations

Leg elevation can set you in *rest and digest* mode by helping you to get relaxed while improving your digestion. The goal of this exercise is to "pull gravitation on digestive organs" (Regan, 2021). It's a simple way to avoid bloating, cramps, and irregular bowel movements. It can strengthen the immune system, release anxiety and headaches, and help to get sleep as well. To get started, take a sitting position facing a wall, with a folded blanket underneath you. Then, lay down your upper body and put your legs up against the wall. Keep your sitz bones away from touching the wall. Keep your legs active. Try to stay in this position for 10 minutes while breathing slowly.

Body Twisting

Body twisting is a combination of breathing and abdominal muscle contractions. This is how you do it. Start with lying on your back. Bend your knees and put your feet on the ground. Next, take a deep breath. Then, focus on your belly button as you try to exhale from your lungs. Make sure to feel your stomach as small as possible.

Biking

It is another exercise to relax your abdominal muscles. It helps to ease digestion by stimulating the digestive tract. Biking is beneficial for the gut as it reduces bloating and irregular bowel movements, while increasing your energy. Precisely, biking can effectively reduce water loss in stools. Besides, it is beneficial to lose belly fat.

STEP-BY-STEP AEROBIC EXERCISES

Aerobic is one of the best physical activities to enhance gut health. Regular practice can also improve cardio-vascular health and lung capacity. Apart from that, it's beneficial to lose weight and gain strength and vitality.

The following exercises include different steps to practice aerobics on your own.

- Basic left and right. It consists of alternating steps between your left and right foot (Cronkleton, 2019). It's simple: Step up with the left foot and step down backward with the right one. Then, you can continue by stepping up with the right foot and stepping down with the left one.

- A-step move. To start, stand next to the bench on your left side (Cronkleton, 2019). Then, step up to the center of the bench with your left foot. Next, lift your right foot to meet the right. Step down and to the opposite by starting with your right foot this time and continue the same process by alternating between your left and right foot.

- Charleston. First, take a step forward with the right foot to the left side of the step. Then, step forward with your left foot and raise your knee. Next, take a step back with your left foot. Finally, step backward and lunge back with your right foot. Continue the same process by alternating between your left and right foot (Cronkleton, 2019).

- Tap up. Stand near a step box and place your feet wider than your shoulder width. Put your right foot on the left side of the step box. Then, tap your left foot on the step box and step down with your left foot. Continue by placing your left foot on the right side of the step box. Tap your right foot on the step box and step down on the floor with your left foot, then the right (Biswas, 2014).

- T Step. Position yourself near a step box. Put your right foot on the step box, then the left.

Step down with your right foot first, followed by your left foot. Alternate between your left and right feet and repeat this 15 times (Biswas, 2014).

- Across the top. Take a step box and put it on your right side. Then, step on the step box with your right foot and step down with your left foot. Do the same with your left foot. Repeat the exercise 20 times.
- Repeater. This exercise consists of putting your left leg on the step box diagonally to the right. Then you use your right leg to kick up while bending your knees. Then alternate between your two legs and repeat the same exercise 15 times (Biswas, 2014).
- Step and Kick. So, put your right foot on the bench and use your left foot to kick in front of you. Then, step back and put your left foot on the bench and kick with your right foot (Biswas, 2014).
- Knee Lift Step. This exercise consists of lifting one of your feet without touching the bench while the other is placed on the bench. Then, step back and repeat the same with the other foot lifted while the one is on the bench (Biswas, 2014).

- Step and Lunge. Place your right foot on the bench and position your knee to 90 degrees. Then, place your left leg behind you. Then, repeat the same process by alternating your left and right foot (Biswas, 2014).

RESISTANCE TRAINING FOR GOOD GUT HEALTH

Leg Adduction

Leg adduction is an important exercise to strengthen your adductors, a group of muscles located on your inner thighs. It offers stability for the lower body. To do it, start by lying on your side and bend your top knee. Next, place your top foot in front of your bottom knee. Then, lift your lower leg off the floor.

Plank

This exercise consists of raising your body up with your toes and elbows so that your chest and abdomen don't touch the floor. Try to be straight and hold on for 10 seconds, then increase to 20 seconds and so forth. Plank is easy to do, yet it can effectively improve digestion and elimination as it helps to stimulate the blood and the abdominal organs.

Side Plank

Side plank is beneficial to maintain core strengths and improve balance. This is the same as plank, but instead, you lie on your side and raise your body up by using your foot and your elbow. Try to hold on for 10 seconds, then increase to 20 seconds and so forth.

Short Arc Squats

To practice this exercise, stand against a wall and put two rolled towels between your knees. Then, slide down the wall to have your knees bent to 60 degrees. Stay in the same position for 10 seconds, then increase to 20 seconds and so forth.

Straight Leg Raises

You can practice straight leg raises by lying on your back and bending your knee. Then, lift your other knee off the floor until your thighs become parallel. Alternate and repeat 10 times.

Wall Shin Raises

For this exercise, start by standing against the wall, lifting your toes towards your body with your weight on your heels. Then, let it down but try not to touch the floor as you will raise it again. Repeat this exercise 10 times with each of your left and right toes.

Heel Step-Downs

The best way to do heel step-downs is to stand with your feet close to each other. Next, take a step forward as you would normally do. Try to keep your heel from flexing down as you move your weight forward. Repeat this exercise 10 times for each side.

Arm Raises

You can practice this exercise by standing straight first. Keep one end of an exercise band under your right foot and the other end with your right hand. Try raising your arm to the side until it is on the same level as your shoulder. Then, hold for five seconds and repeat 10 times. Do the same with your other arm. Next, raise your arm in front of you by leaning on your shoulder. Hold on for five seconds, then slowly lower your arm. Repeat it 10 times and practice the same with the other arm.

External Rotation

For this exercise, put one end of an exercise band on a doorknob and stand sideways on your left while you keep the other end with your right hand. Then, try "to pull the band away from your body with your elbow against your right side." Practice this 10 times.

YOGA-ASANAS FOR GREAT GUT HEALTH

Yoga is a practice to connect the mind with the body to promote health and spiritual enlightenment. Asana means physical practice. Yoga-asanas is then a "combination of movement, breathing techniques, and meditation" (Lederle, 2018). Yoga can influence gut health by helping you to manage stress and improve "physical movement or motility of the gut system." Researchers have found that yoga can be used as a complementary remedy for the treatment of IBS. The following yoga poses are favorable to promote digestion and enhance gut health.

Seated Side Bend or Parsva Sukhasana

This pose can be helpful for digestion, and it can particularly help to reduce bloating and gas (Davidson, 2021). This is how you do it. Take a sitting position with your legs crossed and your arms touching the floor. Then, raise your left arm while leaning on your right side by placing your right forearm on the floor facing outward. Don't forget to inhale and exhale slowly four to five times. Then, switch sides and repeat.

Seated Twist or Ardha Matsyendrasana

This exercise is important to regulate your bowel movements and aids in removing waste through your gut system (Davidson, 2021). Therefore, it should be practiced in the morning before breakfast or six hours after taking a meal. Take a sitting position with your legs stretched out. Next, bend your left leg and place it outside your right knee. Keep your left heel on the floor. Then bend your right knee and put your right heel near your left buttock. Keep this position and breathe four to five times.

Supine Spinal Twist or Supta Matsyendrasana

To start, lie down on your back. Bend your knees and raise your hips off the ground and shift them to the right about one inch (Davidson, 2021). Then, let them back to the floor. Next, place your right knee on your chest. By keeping your left leg straight, gently move your right knee over your left. Then put your right leg on your left one. Keep this position for four to five breaths.

Knees to Chest or Apanasana

This pose helps to stimulate the large intestine and ease bowel movements (Davidson, 2021). To start, lie down on the floor. Bring your knees toward your chest and use your arms to keep them together. Stay in the same position for four to five breaths.

Cat-Cow or Marjaryasana-Bitilasana

To start, put your hands and knees on the floor, mimicking a cat pose (Davidson, 2021). Make sure they are aligned with your shoulders and your hips. Then, try to move down your belly so that your tailbone goes up. Next, raise your head by looking upward. Keep this position for four to five breaths.

Cobra Pose or Bhujangasana

To start, lie on your stomach and bend your elbows and your hands on the floor. Then, try to "touch the floor by extending your feet" (Davidson, 2021). Then, raise your upper body up and forward while keeping your pelvis on the floor. Keep this position for four to five breaths.

Bow Pose or Dhanurasana

Begin this pose by lying on your stomach and raising your feet so they are close to your buttocks (Davidson, 2021). Then, take your ankles and let your knees become wider than your hips. Next, lift your thighs from the floor while maintaining your pelvis on the floor. Hold the same position for four to five breaths.

Belly Twist or Jathara Parivartanasana

Lie on your back and try to shift your hips about an inch to the right. Continue the exercise by raising your feet off the ground while keeping both your knees and feet closer. Try to make a rotation movement with your hips and move your legs to the left while keeping your upper body flat on the floor (Davidson, 2021). Then, put down your legs slowly by leaning on your gravity. Practice this exercise for four to five breaths.

Corpse Pose or Shavasana

This exercise focuses on controlling your breath (Davidson, 2021). Start with lying on your back and keep your arms on your sides. Then, close your eyes and try to take some deep breaths for four seconds, hold them for another four seconds, and count four while you exhale. To avoid distraction and unwelcoming thoughts, keep your attention on your stomach. Practice this exercise for five minutes.

Choosing the right exercises and committing yourself to daily practice can effectively improve your gastrointestinal tract. When you decide to do simple exercises, you are also building healthy habits for your wellbeing. You are training your body to move and relax at the same time. I can't emphasize enough the importance of taking target exercises to enhance your digestion and be free of any pain and discomfort that come with digestive problems. So, start with what's appealing to you the most. Choose the one that feels easy to do for you. Make sure that you are 100% committed to it.

Stick to a schedule and see the transformation you will benefit from it. And if you are not keen on exercising yet, don't hesitate to try yoga asanas as well. Yoga poses can be a little bit challenging to do in the beginning but follow the instructions and explore those different poses. Then, choose what's best for yourself and try to practice every day. What's more, you can also opt for the yoga pose that is related to your treatments and your health conditions. Exercising is something you should be grateful for. If you are able to dedicate even five minutes a day to cultivate your gut-brain-muscle connection, then you are preventing discomfort and problems related to your gut. Therefore, make your decisions and take small steps at a time. And if you ever miss a day or two, don't worry, keep going. You are not trying to be perfect. You are simply striving to get better and feel good in your skin and your gut. In the next chapter, we'll continue the journey with meditation. Why meditation? Why should you meditate? In what manner is meditation beneficial for your gut? How can it release you from the uneasiness of digestive problems? That's what you will find out in the next chapter. Get ready!

8

THE POWER OF BREATH

What is stress? In what conditions do you feel stressed? How is stress related to the gut? Good questions because you're going to discover a new way of living to handle stress and foster your gut health at the same time. You've probably noticed how your gut reacts when you feel hungry or how you have butterflies in your stomach when you are excited about an event or a meeting. Well, these are just the tip of the iceberg because the connection between your brain and your gut is way more impressive than you can imagine. But instead of dwelling on the side effects of stress on the gut, why not tap into the power of stress management to better your gut? Before that, let's talk about the connection between stress and the gut. Above all, stress, or the fight-and-flight response to danger, has always existed in human beings (Atlas Bio Med, 2022). Later, scientists have found out the consequences of such a reaction in the gut. First, when you feel stressed, there is an increase in cortisol production which then impacts your body, including your gut. Second, the effects may differ from one person to another, but the main thing is that's how the brain affects your gut. You might have nausea, or suddenly your appetite disappears, or you have an intense urge to go to the bathroom. But there's more. When your body experiences stress frequently, also called chronic stress, such a situation can induce obesity, eating disorders, heart disease, and depression (Atlas Bio Med, 2022). Furthermore, chronic stress can result in gut inflammation. Fortunately, you can effectively fight stress starting by improving your quality of sleep.

SLEEP AND GUT HEALTH

According to researchers, a lack of sleep is one of the main causes of stress. It means that when you experience sleep deprivation, your body produces more cortisol, the stress hormone. Yet, the more you feel stressed, the higher the risk of gut diseases such as leaky gut syndrome. This is because increased stress influences the intestinal permeability. When the intestine loses its permeability, toxins can access your bloodstream and throughout the body, which then leads to inflammation, bloating, and food sensitivities. Therefore, stress due to the lack of sleep ends up being the cause of an imbalance in gut function. What's more, a lack of sleep can also impact digestive health as it can influence the appetite in a negative way. Have you noticed how hungry you become when you've not slept well during the night? In fact, your first reaction may be to grab some fast and delicious food since your body wants some form of compensation due to the lack of sleep. Yet, we've seen how processed food can negatively impact your gut health. In other words, sleep deprivation does harm your gut in different ways.

MEDITATION

How Meditation Reduces Stress

Meditation is the door to unlocking your peace of mind. When you are stressed out, you have mixed feelings, and you are overwhelmed with mostly negative emotions. Meditation is a way to restore calm, peace, and relaxation in your mind. When you take the time to meditate, you gain more control over your feelings and become a master of your own mind. It means that stress leaves you powerless, while meditation can make you powerful. When you adopt meditation as a habit and a lifestyle, you don't have to resist negative emotions anymore. In fact, the more you meditate, the better you become at feeling peaceful through acceptance. In other words, you are no longer the victim of your negative feelings because you've responded to stress effectively. To gain such a skill, you have to dedicate time to meditation.

Meditation Steps

Did you know that you can achieve a meditative state in different ways? It means that you can choose to practice meditation in the way that is appealing to you the most. Most importantly, you can benefit from meditation instantly, especially when you undergo stressful situations. All you have to do is follow the next steps and get good at practicing them. Whether you are new to meditation or have practiced meditation in the past, you can still manage stress through meditation. In fact, everyone can benefit from meditation and achieve peace of mind. Remember, it's not just your brain that benefits from it; the goal is to take care of your gut health as well.

Breathe Deeply

To start this technique:

1. Get yourself comfortable.
2. Choose clothes that make you feel at ease.

3. Choose a comfortable position by sitting, for example.
4. Straighten your back, close your eyes, and take five seconds to prepare yourself.
5. Take a deep breath through your nose.
6. Hold on for five seconds.
7. Release the air from your nose.
8. During this time, be attentive to how your belly expands the moment you inhale, as you put your left hand on your chest and the right one on your belly. This way, you can feel your belly moving and get totally immersed in the experience. Repeat the same process four to five times.

Scan Your Body

Body Scan is another method to meditate and manage stress. The principle is simple: You focus on each part of your body to relish every feeling you experience now. Start with taking a comfortable position by lying down on a couch, for example. Put your hands on each side of your body. Next, focus on your breathing. Notice how your chest and abdomen are moving for each breath you inhale and exhale. Then, start paying attention to each part of your body. Is there a feeling related to it? Do you feel relaxed, stressed, or in pain? You are free to choose which part of your body to focus on. The goal is to recognize any negative feelings to release them.

Repeat a Mantra

Mantras are words, syllables, or affirmations you repeat saying during a moment of calmness and peace. When it comes to meditation, focus is the key. Therefore, the first thing you should do is to choose a mantra and focus on it. It could be *om*, or *aum, so hum,* or *I am*, etc. Affirmations could be like I am calm, I am powerful, I am capable, I am in control, and so forth. It can be one sentence or more. Next, find a calm place and make sure to get a comfortable position. Once you are settled, set a timer. Determine how long you need and have to practice this session. To get yourself relaxed, control your breathing. Then you can start your mantra. Don't forget to pay attention to what you're saying. Let new thoughts come and go. Don't rush into standing up when your timer goes off. Instead, take a moment to reflect on your feelings and your experience.

Walk and Meditate

Walking meditation is about engaging with yourself while you take a walk. It means that you can learn to be mindful, even if it's just walking in a place you're familiar with. The essential thing is to pay attention to things you've never thought of before, such as your pace, your breath, the way you walk, and the place you are in. To start, it's important to set aside time for practicing. Make sure that you are available as you will take this walk slowly without rushing. Next, notice your movements, your usual thoughts, and your environment. Don't forget to feel your breathing, as this will help you to center your attention on yourself. Welcome any thoughts that come to your mind. Finally, be regular in your walking meditation to benefit from all the advantages of mindfulness. Walking meditation can be helpful when you want to take a break from distressing situations or when you need some time to make some tough decisions. Getting your mind off your current circumstance will boost your focus and clear out your mind.

Engage in Prayer

Prayer is simply the act of talking to God, the Universe, or what you choose to believe. The most important thing is to get your thoughts and your wishes out of your mind. You can pray wherever you are and at any moment of your day. Prayer is effective because it gives a break to your thoughts. Similar to meditation, you direct your mind to focus on yourself. Prayer can be a way to be thankful for your situation and to show your gratitude, but it can also be a way to ask for signs, guidance, or help from God. When you pray, don't strive to be perfect. Talk the way you would talk to a friend. Use your own words. Say what you have in mind. In other, when engaging in prayer, be yourself. When your thoughts wander, acknowledge them. You can say them out loud in your prayer as well. The best way to manage overthinking is to accept your thoughts. Wandering thoughts often occur when you pray, and it's okay. Just acknowledge them.

Read and Reflect

Reading is another way to practice mindfulness and reduce the effects of stress on yourself. To do so, choose a passage or a sentence you want to meditate on. You can opt for any kind of book or content you love or are interested in. Then, reread this sentence or passage three to five times. Next, take a break to think about your reading. Determine your opinions and your thoughts about it. Recognize the emotions you feel at this moment. What does this sentence of passage make you feel? Most importantly, what do you intend to do about it? Is this passage helping you to change something in your life, to act, or open your mind to new things you've never foreseen? After that, say it out loud and use it like a mantra. Finally, take some action. For example, you can end this session with a prayer, or you can list different perspectives and decisions you want to make. You can also craft a simple to-do list or jot down new ideas you've found during this reflection.

Focus on Love and Kindness

Did you know that positive feelings can bring instant happiness and relaxation to your mind? If you are in the middle of a crisis or challenging event, remind yourself of your passion, your love, and anything that you've been proud of. Positive feelings can change your mind and shift your attention from stress to peace of mind. Try this exercise by making a list of the things you love. You can write them down in your notebook or on your phone. Whenever you feel low, stressed, or discouraged, remind yourself to read your list out loud. Another thing you can do is to be compassionate to yourself. Write kind words about yourself: your strengths, your qualities, your skills, your passion, and the things that make you proud of yourself. By being kind to yourself, you give room for positive things to come into your mind. It is especially a way to distract yourself from stress and negativity.

Building Your Meditation Skills

Mindfulness Meditation

Mindfulness meditation aims to bring awareness to your thoughts. What's amazing about mindfulness is that you can go into the state of being mindful in your daily practice. It means that you can access the feeling of peace when you brush your teeth or take a walk or when you take some rest. Once you start paying attention to your thoughts or your inner self-talk, you shed light on your emotions and thought patterns. You can prevent any negative thoughts to affect your mood or your assumptions simply by being mindful. Mindfulness is also helpful to manage stress and anxiety. You can feel stressed in any circumstance. In fact, everyone can get stressed at any moment of their day. However, you can reduce stress by taking care of your emotions. How to do so? Take a break from your activity and listen to your heartbeat, take some deep breaths, and start paying attention to your emotions. Recognize your feelings. Do you feel unloved? Do you feel disappointed? Are you in pain? Are you afraid of something? Do you feel powerless? Whatever you are feeling at this moment, acknowledge it. That's the best way to practice mindfulness and minimize overwhelming emotions.

Now, I want to teach you a simple way to combine mindfulness and meditation for stress relief. The key is to start setting aside a few minutes each day then practice more often as possible whenever you have the time. First, choose a calm place, then take a sitting position or lie down. Get yourself comfortable. Then, relax by taking a breath. Next, direct your attention to this present moment. Listen to the sound around you. Let your thoughts come and go. Don't be resistant. Try to control your breath and notice your environment. Start doing this for five minutes per session.

Spiritual Meditation

Spiritual meditation is a way to *connect with a higher power*, God, or the Universe through meditation, prayer, and self-reflection. When you practice spirituality, you enter the state of being present while feeling the presence of a higher power. It's when you feel one with your God or the Universe. In fact, spiritual meditation is the path to immersing fully in spirituality to strengthen your faith and your beliefs. It also helps to discover and understand your purpose and life's meaning. What does spiritual meditation do with stress? Well, when you surrender yourself to a higher power, you feel at peace and relaxed. You start to let off worries, negativity, and stressful thoughts. As a matter of fact, you can use spiritual meditation as a stress relief if you want to. The choice is up to you. When it comes to spiritual meditation, you don't have to force yourself or put pressure on what you should do. After all, you choose what you believe in. The key is to practice spiritual meditation in the way that suits you the most. You can do it by meditating, for example. You can do so by paying attention to your breath. You can also practice a mantra or a prayer. Or you can simply take a moment alone in a quiet space and choose to feel connected and powerful with a higher power. Assume such a feeling to start seeing changes in your mind and your perspective. Most importantly, when you become good at spiritual meditation, you release tension, become relaxed, and become aware of your inner power.

Focused Meditation

Focused meditation consists of directing your focus on something intentionally and on purpose. It means that you are engaging your attention in the present moment. Focused meditation is easier than classic meditation because your mind has something to concentrate on. You can choose any object of focus for your mind. You can choose to focus on music, an object, a place, an image, or a sound.

Follow these steps for a focused meditation:

- Choose something you want to focus on.
- Sit in a quiet space with a comfortable position.
- Get into a relaxed state by taking some deep breaths, relaxing your shoulders, and thinking of nothing.
- Engage all your senses on the specific object. Listen, touch, watch, and fully experience this moment.

- Don't think about it or analyze it. If any thought comes to your mind, let it come and go. Keep your attention on your target.

Focused meditation is beneficial for improving your concentration and reduce overthinking. It helps you keep your awareness on one thing at a time. In fact, it's the best way to alleviate internal monologue and the tendency to think about different things at the same time. In other words, it creates a moment of peace and extreme focus for your mind.

Movement Meditation

Movement meditation is about relishing the experience of doing an activity. When you are fully attentive to what you're doing, you are practicing meditation. Let's take the example of dancing or walking. When you practice dancing, you pay attention to your movement. You are giving your attention to your move. It means that you are in a meditative state where your senses are fully focused on one thing at a time, in this case, your movement. Movement meditation doesn't have to be a specific activity. It could be writing, massaging, reading, drawing, gardening, or walking. The key to successful practice in this meditation is to focus on your move rather than the goal of the movement. You can do it on purpose regardless of your activity, or you can dedicate a moment to experience it. Start with having some space for yourself where you don't feel distracted. Then, choose an activity you love to do. Now, get relaxed and control your breaths. Next, practice the activity by taking your time. Notice everything and engage all your senses. Finally, pay attention to your feelings at the moment. Focused meditation is about taking the time to slow down and cherish simple moments of your daily life. You don't have to change anything or learn a new activity. You just must embrace your daily life and the things you do and love doing.

Mantra Meditation

Mantra meditation involves repeating a word or an affirmation to increase your awareness. If you struggle to keep your attention on the present moment, using a mantra can be helpful as it offers something for your mind to focus on. In this case, it's the mantra or the affirmation. Common mantra meditation includes the Sanskrit "So Hum," which means I am. So, the first step to practicing mantra meditation is to choose the mantra itself. What's your goal for doing this meditation? Is it to increase your awareness? To silence the voice in your head? To instill positive affirmations or to get relaxed after a stressful day? Choose whatever suits your situation. Then, take a position that gives you comfort during the whole meditation. Don't forget to set a timer. Release the tension by taking some breaths. Now you can recite your mantra out loud. Just like in any similar meditation, your mind may wander. Don't worry. Focus on your mantra instead.

Transcendental Meditation

Developed by Maharishi Mahesh Yogi in the 50s, transcendental meditation consists of repeating a mantra in your head to enhance your awareness of the present moment (Hoshaw, 2020). Keeping your body relaxed is the key. Once you feel relaxed, you can focus on deepening your connection with your inner self. Transcendental meditation doesn't require any specific steps or processes. All you have to do is to get comfortable so that you can relax and concentrate on your mantra. Transcendental meditation is effective because it keeps your mind attentive and conscious. In fact, consciousness is an important part of this type of meditation as if you are able to be fully conscious about yourself, your internal values, and your inner power, you can become the best version of yourself. So, transcendental meditation is essential to be fully conscious of your strengths. What's more, it also helps in reducing stress by using positive affirmations as your mantra. For example, you can remind yourself that you are capable of fighting stress and being peaceful. It helps to alleviate overthinking as well. Once you set your mind on your mantra, you can expel any unnecessary thoughts instantly, and that's the advantage of this type of meditation over classic meditation.

Progressive Meditation

Progressive meditation or body scan consists of raising awareness about how your body feels. It can be used to sense pain, alleviate discomfort, and acknowledge your feelings in a more intentional way. So, progressive meditation involves bringing your attention to each part of your body. Such an experience isn't enough as you will have to get relaxed by managing your breaths in the first place. And this is important because you will only focus on anything except yourself if you don't feel relaxed. Once you have taken some deep breaths, start being attentive to one part of your body. It could be your feet, hands, head, etc. Why not focus on your abdomen, as it's where your gut is? Now, recognize any sensation related to this part of your body. Honestly, how do you feel? Name it, get the word out, and acknowledge the sensation. What's the most important thing about this meditation? It's the fact that you learn to acknowledge your pain, your discomfort, and uneasiness. Instead of saying no to pain, say yes to recognize it. It's the same as with negative emotions. You end up lessening the power of these emotions once you recognize them. Don't forget to breathe to release tension and get relaxed. Research has found that this type of meditation doesn't stop the pain, but it changes the way you see and feel about the pain. Once you change your perspective about what you are feeling, you open your mind to healing. After, pain comes with a feeling, right? In this case, we nurture the feeling to soothe the pain.

Loving-Kindness Meditation

Loving-kindness meditation is a type of meditation that involves creating positive feelings through mindfulness and self-awareness. This is a super simple meditation, and I'm sure you've already done it at least once in your life. Choose a person that you cherish the most in your life (Greater Good in Action, n.d.). Then, imagine how this person makes you feel happy and joyful. Hold a vivid image of the things that this person makes you feel. Think about the attention they give to you. Choose to be grateful to have this person in your life. While you envision all these scenarios, relish this experience by taking some deep breaths. It's important that you feel at ease, undistracted and comfortable when you do this exercise. Now, imagine the expression of love, compassion, and gratitude that you want for this person. Think about the positive things that you want to happen in their lives. Wish them to be fully happy, fulfilled, and at peace with themselves. In fact, return the favor by desiring the person to feel the same as you do now. Send love to them. During this time, if you get distracted, it's okay. Bring back your attention to yourself by feeling your breaths. Then, recultivate the positive emotions that you are feeling about this person and how you want to give them back. Loving-kindness meditation is powerful because it deepens your connection with your loved ones. Most importantly, it fosters acceptance, gratitude, and compassion. Taking the time to nurture your feelings is important to recognize that there's more to life than stress and pain. In fact, everyone has a person that they hold dearly in their heart. When you take the time to practice this exercise, you will know that you are valued, loved, and cherished.

Visualization Meditation

Visualization meditation is a type of meditation that uses the power of imagination to cultivate inner peace and relaxation. It consists of visualizing yourself in the state that you wish to be or in a scenario where you feel positive emotions, such as peace of mind, gratitude, fulfillment, compassion, abundance, and so forth. Beforehand, determine what you wish to achieve from this exercise. Set a goal for yourself: Do you want to feel confident? Do you desire your dreams to unfold? Do you aim to release stress, tension, and negativity?

Once you are sure about your intent for this meditation, let's get started. Similar to any type of meditation, choose a comfortable position. You can lie down or sit. The essential thing is that you are comfortable to practice this exercise. Okay? Next, close your eyes and let your body relax. Enjoy the calmness of the space. Notice your heartbeat. Take control of your breaths. Inhale, then hold your breath for four seconds and exhale. Repeat the same process until you feel completely satisfied. Now, imagine yourself in a place you love the most. Visualize yourself sitting somewhere. Envision how you feel radiant, positive, and grateful in that scenario. If you have a specific goal to reach, then imagine yourself feeling happy with your goal fulfilled. Relish the feeling of pride in your heart. Take into account how your wish is possible because of your power and your strengths. And if your desire is to achieve peace of mind, then picture yourself lying somewhere with no worries or fear. Imagine how relaxed you are at this time. Try to include a mantra that is related to your specific goal. Then, repeat the same mantra in your head. When you do this exercise, use a timer. Visualization meditation is a tool to imagine the best version of yourself and with which you create your self-image and identity. Using your imagination can give you a feeling of power and mastery over your life as you can realize that whatever positive feelings you wish to cultivate, you can do so through your imagination.

BREATHING EXERCISES

Five Deep Breaths

Five deep breaths are a combination of breathing exercises and mantra meditation. The first breath consists of preparing your mind by managing your breath. Take a deep breath and exhale slowly. In the second one, try to inhale and then exhale along with gratitude affirmations such as *I am proud of myself, I am a strong person,* and *I am a capable person.* In the third breath, repeat the same breathing exercise, but this time, focus on affirming your goals and what you want to be today, such as *I want to be brave, I want to be productive,* and *I want to be patient.* In your fourth breath, practice the same breathing exercise and use affirmations about your ideal self, such as *I am compassionate, I am honest,* and *I am abundant.* Finally, on your fifth breath, take a deep breath and get relaxed.

Finger Breathing

Finger breathing is a simple breathing exercise to monitor your breathing and practice mindfulness (Sutton, 2021). This is how you do it. Use your pointer finger to trace the other hands, starting with your thumb. On the way up, inhale. On the way down, exhale. Repeat the same process for each finger. Then, practice the same exercise with the other hand.

4-7-8 Breathing

Developed by Dr. Andrew Weil, 4-7-8 breathing is a powerful breathing exercise to achieve deep relaxation and help to fall asleep (Sutton, 2021). Start by taking a deep breath through your nose for four seconds with a closed mouth. Then, hold your breath for seven seconds. Next, try to breathe out for eight seconds. Repeat the same exercise four times and at least twice a day to gain effective results.

Belly Breathing

Belly breathing, or diaphragmatic breathing, consists of bringing your focus to the movement of your belly while you inhale and exhale. It helps to establish regular breathing, while negative emotions such as stress often force you to take shallow and irregular breaths in an unconscious way. To practice belly breathing, get yourself comfortable by lying down and bending your knees so that your feet stay on the floor. Then, put your hands on top of each other on your abdomen. Close your eyes, breathe in, and breathe out through your nose. Notice how your belly expands and retracts during this time.

Box Breathing

Box breathing is a breathing technique that helps to restore quietness and peace of mind after stressful experiences. This is quite simple, and you can effectively practice it at home or in your office. You can do this by sitting comfortably and putting your feet on the ground. Place your hands on your chest and your lower abdomen. Now, close your eyes, feel your stomach moving, and start breathing in for four seconds. Hold your breath for another four seconds, exhale for four seconds, and finally hold for four seconds. Repeat the same exercise three times.

I invite you instead to take one step at a time. Choose the type of exercise you want to apply, or that seems easy for you, whether it's breathing technique or meditation. The goal of this chapter is to make you aware that you have as many options as you can imagine when it comes to improving your well-being. You can better yourself right now if you want to. All it takes is practice, as one single practice can change your mind, and set you on the path to combat stress. It is possible to repair your gut by fighting stress. It is totally feasible to balance your life by choosing the right foods, the right exercises, and the right practice. All that matters is your choice. I recognize there's a lot to digest, though. There's a lot of information, advice, and practices in this chapter. That's why, in the next chapter, you learn to practice a gut-friendly lifestyle with tools such as journaling and shopping lists. For you have a balanced diet and lifestyle, you have to learn to do so, right? And that's the goal of the next chapter, to help you put into practice everything you've read in this book, and to set you on the right path to change.

STEP 4: LIVING A GUT-FRIENDLY LIFESTYLE

9

THE GUT-CLEANSE JOURNALING

WHAT IS JOURNALING?

Journaling involves writing. It is the act of putting your thoughts, your impression, and your perspectives on paper. It's the way to externalize your feelings, your pain, and the sensation that you feel. It is also a tool with which you manifest your idea, your intention, and your vision in your real life. For example, if you are thinking about starting a meditation or eating more fiber-rich food, then journaling is the tool you use to write your commitments and follow through with them. Consider journaling as something that helps you become a better version of yourself and achieve your different goals.

HOW CAN JOURNALING IMPROVE YOUR GUT HEALTH?

If there is one thing that you need apart from this book, it's a diary or a notebook. First, it's the place where you're going to pay attention to your diet. It's understandable to forget about your health goals when you undergo stress or challenges in life. When you are feeling low emotionally, all you want to eat is what your mind *wants* you to eat. In fact, that's totally natural and normal. Notice how you crave sugar or fast food when you are stressed. That's totally okay. However, you still need to pay attention to your diet because your gut health matters, right? And your weight-loss goal matters as well. That's where journaling can help you. In this notebook, you will take notes about your food intolerances, your allergies, your meal plan, and so forth. Let's admit it; there's nothing more effective than a planned life. Having goals is one thing. Realizing them is another thing. When it comes to removing any obstacles to your gut health, you must plan your diet. With journaling, you have more power over what you eat. What's more, you become aware of the effects of food on your gut and your overall health. Second, journaling is helpful in balancing your lifestyle. We all recognize that exercising is important, but it's easier said than done, right? That's why journaling can assist you in implementing your new habits. It starts with writing your commitments to practice gentle moves that target your digestive health. Then it continues with keeping notes of the best ways you can practice meditation when you feel stressed. Third, you will use journaling to write your own feedback about every change you have experienced in your health, your feelings, and your habits. Consider it as the place where you give your opinions about one specific yoga pose and how another one is more effective for you. Why do you need to do all of that? Changes take time. Getting better gut health in the long term takes time. Hence, you have to invest both your efforts and your time to follow through on your goals. You have to take the time to *care* about your well-being, and the best tool you can use is writing in a journal.

PRACTICING A GUT-CLEANSE JOURNALING

Elimination Phase Journaling

During the elimination phase, use your journal and start writing down your goals. What are your expectations at this stage? If you want to eliminate toxins, write that down. If you want to eat more antioxidant foods, that's fine. The essential thing is to have your goal within your reach. Next, take notes of the best types of food you need to include in your diet. You can always refer to this book and write the foods that are easy for you to prepare. Also, keep track of your meal plan ideas. You can get some inspiration from the suggested meal plans, but you can also have yours. Lastly, write your impression at the end of the day. What are your feelings about this new diet? As you might not be familiar with a gut-friendly diet yet, writing your feedback is important once you make the decision to choose the types of food you want to prioritize, and the ones you want to remove from your diet.

Restoration Phase Journaling

In the restoration phase, you're going to feed your gut with the right food. But first, write down your goals for this step. For example, *I want to feed my inner garden with the right food. I want to diversify my gut microbiota. I want to ease my digestion.* At this stage, you will better understand how certain foods are good for your gut health while others are not. Next, jot down the list of foods you need to prioritize. These include fiber-rich food and probiotics. If you choose to take supplements, that's fine. The key is to restore your gut health with the right foods. Now, take notes of how your body— your gut—reacts to this new diet. Most importantly, how do you feel? Do you notice any improvement in your digestion? Don't forget to write your feedback about this phase.

Reintroduction Phase Journaling

During the reintroduction phase, the essential thing is to keep track of your food reactions as you will finally reintroduce new foods to your diet. These are mostly the ones that don't directly improve your gut health, but you need them to get other health benefits or just because you love them. Start with writing your goal for this step. Do you want to eat some fast food? Fine, write it. Would you love to make some treats and eat sugary foods? That's okay as well. But here's how journaling is going to be helpful to keep your balanced diet: Include your health goals, such as improving your digestion or eating more high-fiber foods. Having in mind your wants and your needs is important to help you make decisions each day to obtain a balanced diet. Once you are aware of your goals while acknowledging your cravings, it will be easier for you to plan your meal and diversify your diet without neglecting your favorite meals.

The R.E.S.T.O.R.E is effective on one condition: You apply it. When it comes to changing your well-being and transforming your life, your intentions and actions matter. With the power of journaling, you can have both. In fact, journaling keeps your mind focused on your goals and helps you monitor your efforts and your commitments. If there is one key actor to make things happen, it's you. You make things happen, and you have the tools to revamp your well-being from now on. In the next chapter, we'll get more practical to help you make healthier food choices and balance your diet. Consider it as the step you will start making changes for your health. After all, food is important for your health. It's crucial to make mindful choices to implement new shopping habits, eat the best foods for your gut, and improve your life on the way.

10

THE GUT-FRIENDLY SHOPPING GIST

WHAT YOU SHOULD HAVE IN YOUR KITCHEN

Below is the list of what you should have in your kitchen to implement new healthy habits.

- Extra-virgin olive oil. This is super healthy, and it's the best oil you can choose if you want to better your health and your gut. It contains antioxidants and is an excellent choice to fight inflammation.
- Greek yogurt. Greek yogurt is rich in probiotics and calcium. You can have it in your breakfast or as a snack. That's why it's a good choice to have it within your reach.

- Honey. Honey is a gut-friendly food. It is a great source of digestive enzymes which are important to ensure digestion. It can replace refined sugar to sweeten your food as well.
- Garlic. Is garlic good for the gut? Yes. Not only does it prevent inflammation, but it also helps to regulate your bowel movements. In fact, garlic is one of the best sources of prebiotics.
- Quinoa. Quinoa has multiple benefits for your health. It is a great source of protein and is naturally gluten-free.

THE BEST PROBIOTICS YOU NEED TO HAVE

Below is a list of probiotic sources you should prioritize over anything else.

- Probiotic yogurt. Probiotic yogurt is excellent for digestion and contains good bacteria, which are essential for your gut health. You can have two servings per day to gain all these benefits.
- Pickles. Pickles have multiple benefits for health as they are rich in antioxidants and probiotics.
- Cottage cheese. Fermented cottage cheese is definitely one of the best gut-friendly foods.

You can have it in your main meals or as a snack. What's more, it's super nutritious and rich in calcium.

- Kefir. This is the best gut-friendly drink you should have in your kitchen. Kefir helps to lessen digestive problems and strengthen bone health.
- Sauerkraut. Sauerkraut is rich in nutrition, such as fiber, vitamins, and minerals. It is also a fermented food, which means that it contains friendly bacteria for your gut.

THE BEST SOURCES OF NATURAL PREBIOTICS TO SHOP

Here are the best prebiotics sources for your gut health.

- Apples. Apples are fiber-rich foods and help to reduce appetite as eating apples gives a sensation of fullness. Besides, they contain antioxidants and prevent the risk of chronic diseases such as obesity, diabetes, and cancer.
- Bananas. Bananas are extremely nutritious and provide different benefits for your health. Rich in nutrients, bananas are a source of energy and beneficial for your heart health and blood

pressure. In addition to that, they help digestion.

- Flaxseed. Eating flaxseed supports digestive health by enhancing digestion and alleviating constipation. It also aids in reducing the risk of heart disease.
- Barley. Rich in fiber, barley is excellent for the gut. Eating barley can help you lessen the feeling of hunger and lose weight.
- Asparagus. Asparagus has antioxidant properties and supports gut health. It is rich in vitamins and can help you balance your weight as well.

A lifestyle change starts with small steps. Having superfoods in your kitchen is helpful for keeping a balanced diet, as it will give you more control over your meal plan. Of course, preparing your meal at home is always the best option. But if your schedule or your work doesn't allow you to do it often, it's still beneficial to have these foods at home. Besides, such an investment will keep you focused on your health goals. Don't hesitate to explore different options and take some inspiration from the suggested foods in the previous chapters. To achieve a gut-friendly lifestyle, keep in mind that you don't have to be too hard on yourself.

Focus on having some of these superfoods in your diet from time to time and minimize processed food as much as possible. Most importantly, being healthy has nothing to do with being perfect in your meal plans. Don't hesitate to explore different diets to find the one that suits you the most.

You're about to embark on a lifestyle change you'll never look back from – and you're in the perfect position to help someone else set out on their own journey.

Simply by sharing your honest opinion of this book and a little about your own experience, you'll show new readers where they can find all the guidance they need to repair their digestive health.

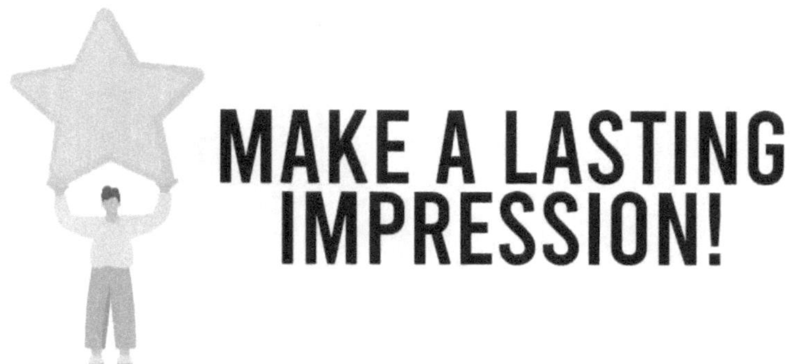

Thank you so much for your support. It's amazing how much impact we can have when we work together.

CONCLUSION

You don't have to be a gut expert to repair your digestive health. If there's one single piece of advice to improve your gut, here it is: Eat more gut-friendly foods and eat less processed foods. However, understanding how your gut works gives you more power over your well-being. Therefore, we've taken the time to explore the different facets of the gut system. First of all, a better eating habit comes with understanding how your body processes food. For example, your gut microbiome ensures the function of your digestive health while your digestive enzymes are your ally to break down foods. Once you are aware of the power of foods in your diet, you will start to comprehend how certain foods are beneficial for your gut while others could be harmful to your overall well-being.

Talking about the gut always includes food and diet. As a matter of fact, if you want to reduce inflammation and the discomfort of digestive problems, processed foods and sugary foods should be avoided. But there's more. You need to consider psychological factors such as stress and sleep if you want to create a healthier gastrointestinal tract. Indeed, the gut and brain are connected. For instance, stress affects your digestive health inducing reactions such as nausea, diarrhea, and loss of appetite, whereas digestive problems can worsen stress and anxiety. Here comes the R.E.S.T.O.R.E method, the path to healing your gut and shifting to a healthier lifestyle. This 3-day gut cleanse process includes the elimination phase, the restoration phase, and the reintroduction phase. It takes into account the natural process of digestive health by removing toxins and stress while feeding your gut with the right foods. What's more, it teaches you to be aware of food intolerances and allergies to better handle your gut system.

A lifestyle change goes hand in hand with a balanced diet. Optimizing the brain-gut-muscle connection is the secret to creating lasting change for your health. It starts with stimulating digestion with the right exercises, such as yoga, aerobics, and biking. With daily practice, you can prevent digestive problems and improve your well-being. What's more, taking care of your gut also means reducing stress. With the help of meditation and breathing exercises, it's possible to alleviate the effects of stress and foster your emotional well-being. Furthermore, being mindful about your food choices will make a difference in your health. As a matter of fact, journaling can help you monitor your diet and implement changes in your lifestyle. Setting health goals and keeping track of your food reactions are important to build a healthier lifestyle. Most importantly, being mindful means listening to your body's needs without neglecting your food preferences. In addition to that, you can leverage the power of journaling during your 3-day gut cleanse process to have a more intimate connection with your gut and your body. But what happens when you've successfully finished your gut cleanse process? Well, don't strive to be perfect or rigid about your diet. Instead, have superfoods in your kitchen to better control your meal plan. It will also help you to diversify your diet without saying *no* to your favorite meals.

It's 100% possible to enhance your well-being with the right method. The key is to be consistent in making small investments each day, whether it's through exercising or eating gut-friendly food. Keep in mind that your efforts will always pay off. Start with small steps at a time. Choose the best activity that is easy for you to start. Engage your senses through mindfulness to control your mood. Make sure that you are enjoying your gut-friendly lifestyle. Don't hesitate to keep learning about the gut to deepen your knowledge and understanding of how it works. If you have the intention to take food supplements, that's fine, but always consider your expectations and your health conditions. Most importantly, be moderate in your diet. Too many probiotics and high-fiber foods are harmful to your health. Therefore, strive to vary your food choices. If you have loved this book and enjoyed your reading experience, please leave a review to inspire others to explore their gut health and say goodbye to inflammation and digestive problems for good.

IMPORTANCE OF HUMAN WORK-OUT

When it comes to health and feeling fine
There's one thing to be done at all times
Rise up and move, and break a sweat
You will not regret it, you may bet
Workout helps and heals the body
Makes you feel good, never shoddy

From head to toe, it does its part
To keep you strong and full of heart
At first it might be tough to start
But once you do, you'll play your part
In staying fit and feeling great
Like a champ, you'll dominate

Your muscles will grow, your heart will pump
Your energy levels will never slump
You'll have more focus, less stress too
And sleep like a baby, it's all true
So don't be lazy, get on the floor
Or hit the gym, and so much more

Find what you like doing, and do it perfectly
Your body will surely thank you, can't you
   tell?
There's running, swimming, lifting weights
Or yoga, Pilates, and cycling rates
Zumba, dance, and martial arts
Or hiking, climbing, playing darts

Whatever you choose, just do it right
Listen to your body, and take flight
Challenge yourself, but don't overdo
Take breaks, drink water, and eat clean too
Remember, workout is not a chore
It's a lifestyle, and so much more

It's a way to show your body love
And to the world, shine like a dove
With each day that passes by
You'll feel like you can touch the sky
Staying active keeps you going
For as long as forever, it's worth knowing

So here's a rhyme to remind you
That working out is key to feel anew
Keep moving and sweating, don't be shy
Your body will thank you, it's no lie!

— MCGRICA, 2023

ABOUT THE AUTHOR

Candi Mcgrica is a health and wellness expert with a passion for gut health. As a child, she struggled with digestive issues, which led to a lifelong fascination with the human digestive system and the role it plays in overall health. After years of struggling with various digestive disorders, she decided to take matters into their own hands and began researching the latest findings on gut health. Through extensive reading and experimentation with their own diet and lifestyle, she was able to alleviate their symptoms and achieve a new level of health and vitality.

Through this book, Candi Mcgrica wants to share her knowledge and experience with others who are struggling with digestive issues. She believes that everyone deserves to live a life free from the discomfort and pain of digestive disorders and hopes that this book will provide readers with the tools and knowledge they need to achieve optimal gut health.

With Candi Mcgrica's personal experience and expertise as your guide, you'll be able to make the necessary changes to your diet and lifestyle to achieve optimal gut health and live your best life.

GLOSSARY

Celiac disease: A gastrointestinal condition brought on by gluten malabsorption.

Leaky gut: A condition when poisons are absorbed by the gut and then enter the bloodstream.

Short-chain fatty acids: The outcome of fiber in the colon being fermented by bacteria.

REFERENCES

Ajmera, R. (2020, September 22). *8 fermented foods and drinks you should try, from kefir to kimchi.* Healthline. https://www.healthline.com/nutrition/8-fermented-foods#8.-Probiotic-yogurt

Aliouche, H. (2022, February 5). *What are the effects of artificial sweeteners on gut health?* News-Medical.net. https://www.news-medical.net/health/What-are-the-Effects-of-Artificial-Sweeteners-on-Gut-Health.aspx#:~:text=Alterations%20in%20the%20gut%20microbiota

Are environmental toxins disrupting your microbiome? (2017, November 15). Lavage Wellness Center. https://lavagewellness.com/environmental-toxins-disrupting-microbiome/#:~:text=Disruption%20to%20the%20microbiome%20by

Aswell, S. (2018, January 29). *Fiber diet: How it changes your gut and how to eat more.* Healthline. https://www.healthline.com/health/food-nutrition/fiber-diet-good-for-gut-and-health#the-verdict-on-fiber

Bagchi, T. (2014). Traditional food & modern lifestyle: Impact of probiotics. *The Indian Journal of Medical Research, 140*(3), 333–335. https://www.ncbi.nlm.nih.gov/pmc/articles/PMC4248377/

Bell, B. (2016, December 8). *Does gluten cause leaky gut syndrome?* Healthline. https://www.healthline.com/nutrition/gluten-leaky-gut#:~:text=Gluten%20causes%20significant%20health%20concerns%20in%20individuals%20with%20an%20intolerance

Biswas, C. (2014, October 21). *Step aerobics: 10 workouts, benefits, and tips.* Stylecraze. https://www.stylecraze.com/articles/benefits-of-step-aerobics-for-weight-loss/

Celiac disease. (2021). Merriam-Webster.com. https://www.merriam-webster.com/dictionary/celiac%20disease

Chai, C. (n.d.). *Why exercise is good for gut health.* EverydayHealth.com. https://www.everydayhealth.com/fitness/can-exercise-boost-my-gut-health/

Constipation (2019). University of Rochester Medical center. https://www.urmc.rochester.edu/encyclopedia/content.aspx?content typeid=85&contentid=p00363

Cronkleton, E. (2019, May 24). *Step aerobics: Benefits, moves, and tips.* Healthline. https://www.healthline.com/health/step-aerobics

Davani-Davari, D., Negahdaripour, M., Karimzadeh, I., Seifan, M., Mohkam, M., Masoumi, S., Berenjian, A., & Ghasemi, Y. (2019). Prebiotics: Definition, types, sources, mechanisms, and clinical applications. *Foods, 8*(3), 92.

Davidson, K. (2021, February 9). *Can yoga help aid digestion? 9 poses to try.* Healthline. https://www.healthline.com/nutrition/yoga-posture-for-digestion#The-bottom-line

Elmagd, M. (2016). Benefits, need and importance of daily exercise. *International Journal of Physical Education, Sports and Health, 3*(5), 22–27. http://www.kheljournal.com/archives/2016/vol3issue5/PartA/3-4-55-201.pdf

Felson, S. (2017, January 26). *What are probiotics?* WebMD. https://www.webmd.com/digestive-disorders/what-are-probiotics

Fields, L. (2010, November 3). *How fiber helps your digestive health.* WebMD. https://www.webmd.com/diet/features/fiber-digestion

5 exercises that aid in optimal digestive health. (2022, May 18). Allied Digestive Health. https://allieddigestivehealth.com/5-exercises-that-aid-in-optimal-digestive-health/

5 superfoods for those on a detox diet. (2023). Wellbeingnutrition.com. https://wellbeingnutrition.com/blogs/listing/5-superfoods-for-those-on-a-detox-diet

Food allergy - symptoms and causes. (2017). Mayo Clinic. https://www.mayoclinic.org/diseases-conditions/food-allergy/symptoms-causes/syc-20355095

Griffin, R. M. (n.d.). *Fiber for heart and digestive health.* WebMD. https://www.webmd.com/vitamins-and-supplements/supplement-guide-fiber

Fiber. (2018, June 6). Harvard School of Public Health. https://www.hsph.harvard.edu/nutritionsource/carbohydrates/fiber/

Hoshaw, C. (2020, September 17). *Which type of meditation is right for you?* Healthline. https://www.healthline.com/health/mental-health/types-of-meditation#visualization-meditation

How stress impacts the microbiome and gut health. (2022, May 14). Atlas Biomed Blog |Atlas Bio Med. https://atlasbiomed.com/blog/how-stress-impacts-the-gut-via-the-gut-brain-axis/

Ianiro, G., Pecere, S., Giorgio, V., Gasbarrini, A., & Cammarota, G. (2016). Digestive enzyme supplementation in gastrointestinal diseases. *Current Drug Metabolism, 17*(2), 187–193. https://doi.org/10.2174/138920021702160114150137

Iliades, C. (2015, June 25). *4 essential vitamins for digestive health.* EverydayHealth.com. https://www.everydayhealth.com/digestive-health/essential-vitamins-for-digestive-health.aspx

Iliades, C. (2018, October 16). *How stress affects digestion.* EverydayHealth.com. https://www.everydayhealth.com/wellness/united-states-of-stress/how-stress-affects-digestion/

Jane, M. (2016, April 2). *How short-chain fatty acids affect health and weight.* Healthline. https://www.healthline.com/nutrition/short-chain-fatty-acids-101

Kinsinger, S. (2017, June 7). *How your brain and emotions control your gut.* Loyola Medicine. https://www.loyolamedicine.org/about-us/blog/how-your-brain-and-emotions-control-your-gut

Lawrence, K., & Hyde, J. (2017). Microbiome restoration diet improves digestion, cognition and physical and emotional wellbeing. *PLOS ONE, 12*(6), e0179017. https://doi.org/10.1371/journal.pone.0179017

Leaky gut syndrome. (2022b, April 6). Cleveland Clinic. https://my.clevelandclinic.org/health/diseases/22724-leaky-gut-syndrome

Lederle, D. (2018, June 18). *Yoga for digestion.* The Healthy Maven. https://www.thehealthymaven.com/YOGA-FOR-DIGESTION/

Loving-Kindness meditation. (n.d.). Ggia.berkeley.edu. https://ggia.berkeley.edu/index.php/practice/loving_kindness_meditation

Manaker, L. (2021, November 19). *How does deep breathing improve your digestion?* Verywell Health. https://www.verywellhealth.com/diaphragmatic-breathing-stress-digestion-5209648

Mcgrica, C. (2023, April). *Importance of Human Work-Out.*

Migala, J. (2015, February 16). *The health benefits of water.* EverydayHealth.com. https://www.everydayhealth.com/water-health/water-body-health.aspx

Moore, W. (n.d.). *Which probiotic is right for you?* WebMD. https://www.webmd.com/digestive-disorders/pick-right-probiotic

Mudge, L. (2022, March 29). *What is gut health and why is it important?* Livescience.com. https://www.livescience.com/what-is-gut-health-and-why-is-it-important

Nagy-Szakal, D., Williams, B. L., Mishra, N., Che, X., Lee, B., Bateman, L., Klimas, N. G., Komaroff, A. L., Levine, S., Montoya, J. G., Peterson, D. L., Ramanan, D., Jain, K., Eddy, M. L., Hornig, M., & Lipkin, W. I. (2017). Fecal metagenomic profiles in subgroups of patients with myalgic encephalomyelitis/chronic fatigue syndrome. *Microbiome, 5*(1). https://doi.org/10.1186/s40168-017-0261-y

Pattemore, C. (2020, October 14). *Just the facts: Gut health.* Greatist. https://greatist.com/discover/facts-gut-health#dietary-tips

Pietrangelo, A. (2020, February 28). *What are digestive enzymes and how do they work?* Healthline. https://www.healthline.com/health/exocrine-pancreatic-insufficiency/the-role-of-digestive-enzymes-in-gi-disorders#how-they-work

Powell Key, A. (2021, November 29). *What are digestive enzymes?* WebMD. https://www.webmd.com/diet/what-are-digestive-enzymes

Probiotics: What is it, benefits, side effects, food & types. (2020, March 9). Cleveland Clinic. https://my.clevelandclinic.org/health/articles/14598-probiotics

Regan, S. (2021, June 18). *Feeling bloated? This simple exercise could offer some relief.* Mindbodygreen. https://www.mindbodygreen.com/articles/legs-up-the-wall-pose

Sanders, B. (2019, June 19). *Fermented foods for gut health.* UMass Chan Medical School. https://www.umassmed.edu/nutrition/blog/blog-posts/2019/6/fermented-foods-for-gut-health/

Seriously delicious detox salad. (2017, January 6). Gimme Some Oven. https://www.gimmesomeoven.com/seriously-delicious-detox-salad/

7 detox vitamins & minerals that rid the body of toxins. (2023, April 5). The Recovery Village at Palmer Lake. https://www.palmerlakerecovery. com/resources/7-detox-vitamins-minerals-rid-body-toxins/

7 Signs of a Healthy Gut + Tips To Improve Digestive Health (2022, June 16). Www.everlywell.com. https://www.everlywell.com/blog/food-allergy/signs-of-healthy-gut/

Simpson, K. (2020, June 7). *Sleep and digestion - how to improve your gut health.* Sleep Advisor. https://www.sleepadvisor.org/sleep-and-digestion/

Sutton, J. (2021, December 20). *7 stress-relief breathing exercises for calming your mind.* PositivePsychology.com. https://positivepsychol ogy.com/breathing-exercises-for-stress-relief/

The bacterial challenge: Time to react A call to narrow the gap between multidrug-resistant bacteria in the EU and the development of new antibacterial agents. (n.d.). http://www.ema.europa.eu/documents/ report/bacterial-challenge-time-react_en.pdf

The Brain-Gut Connection. (2019). John Hopkins Medicine. https:// www.hopkinsmedicine.org/health/wellness-and-prevention/the-brain-gut-connection

The central role of the gut. (n.d.). Danone Research & Innovation. https:// www.danoneresearch.com/gut-and-microbiology/the-central-role-of-the-gut/

The gut-brain connection. (2019, April 19). Harvard Health. https://www. health.harvard.edu/diseases-and-conditions/the-gut-brain-connection

The rise of digestive diseases and how to take control of your gut health. (n.d.). BodyBio. https://bodybio.com/blogs/blog/digestive-diseases-on-rise

38 Hippocrates Quotes About Health, Food And Medicine >. (2020, August 8). Wise Owl Quotes. https://wiseowlquotes.com/ hippocrates/

Tiffany. (2019, January 4). *Best simple tossed green salad.* Creme de La Crumb. https://www.lecremedelacrumb.com/best-simple-tossed-green-salad/

Tresca, A. (2022, October 24). *Which fiber supplement is right for you?*

Verywell Health. https://www.verywellhealth.com/before-you-buy-fiber-supplements-1941633#:~:text=Fiber%20supplements%20can%20be%20used

Villines, Z. (2017, July 29). *Free radicals: How do they affect the body?* Www.medicalnewstoday.com. https://www.medicalnewstoday.com/articles/318652

What are prebiotics and what do they do? (2022a, March 14). Cleveland Clinic. https://health.clevelandclinic.org/what-are-prebiotics/

Wu, J., Zhang, Y., Ye, L., & Wang, C. (2021). The anti-cancer effects and mechanisms of lactic acid bacteria exopolysaccharides in vitro: A review. *Carbohydrate Polymers, 253*, 117308. https://doi.org/10.1016/j.carbpol.2020.117308

Zhang, Y.-J., Li, S., Gan, R.-Y., Zhou, T., Xu, D.-P., & Li, H.-B. (2015). Impacts of gut bacteria on human health and diseases. *International Journal of Molecular Sciences, 16*(12), 7493–7519. https://doi.org/10.3390/ijms16047493

Zinöcker, M., & Lindseth, I. (2018). The western diet–microbiome-host interaction and its role in metabolic disease. *Nutrients, 10*(3), 365. https://doi.org/10.3390/nu10030365

Zoppi, L. (2021, March 30). *Detoxing foods: What are they? What are the benefits?* Www.medicalnewstoday.com. https://www.medicalnewstoday.com/articles/detoxing-foods#pulses

Zucchini frittata. (n.d.). Eating Well. https://www.eatingwell.com/recipe/248685/zucchini-frittata/